Rejuvenating Skin Without Surgery

MARIO LUCA RUSSO, MD

WITH PHILIPPA PIGACHE

FOREWORD BY TINA ALSTER, MD

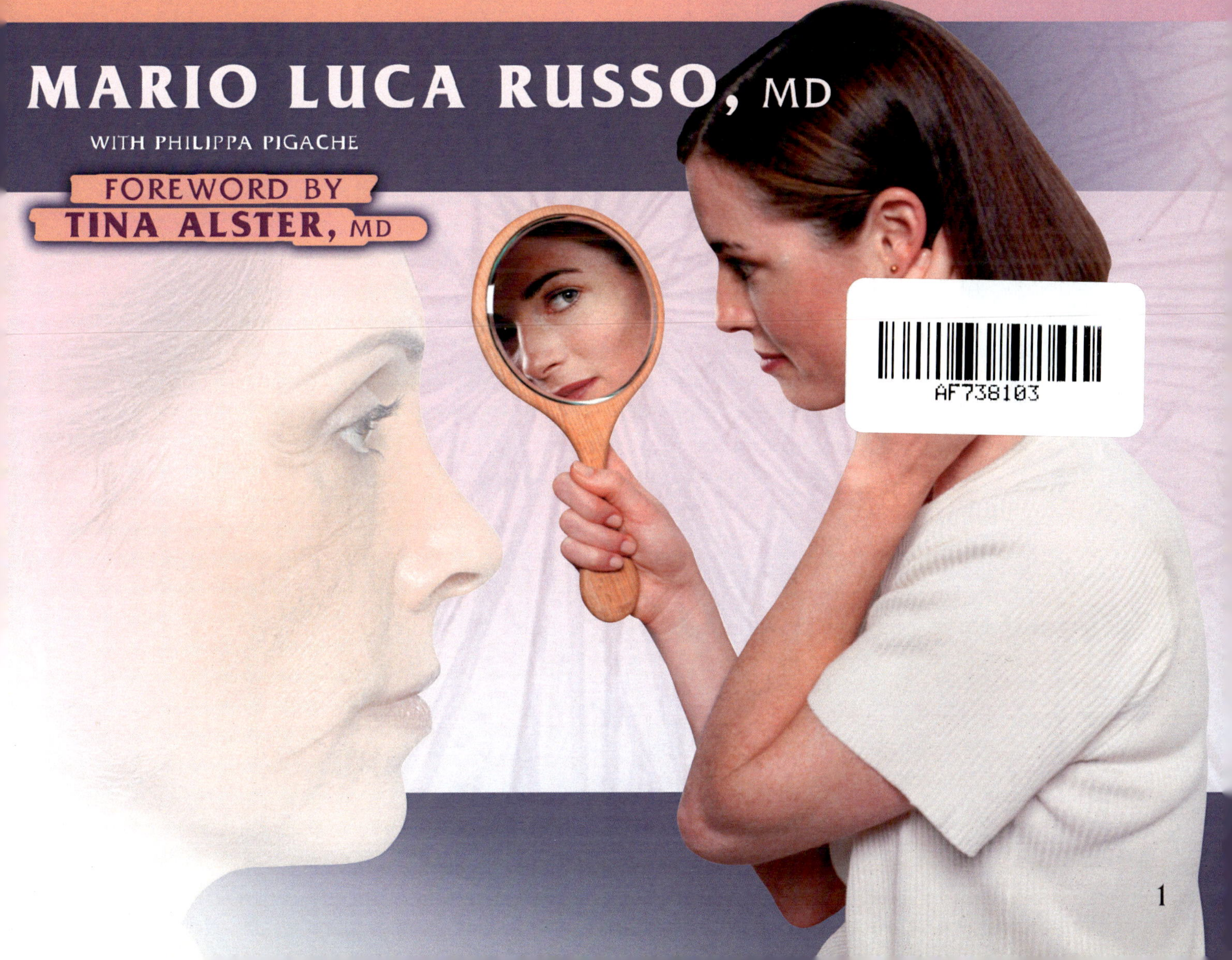

ISBN: 978-1-873413-94-4

Rejuvenating Skin Without Surgery

MARIO LUCA RUSSO, MD

WITH PHILIPPA PIGACHE

Merit Publishing International

North American address:
1095 Jupiter Park Drive,
Suite 7,
Jupiter, FL 33458,
USA

Tel: 561 697 1116

European address:
50 Highpoint,
Heath Road,
Weybridge, Surrey, KT13 8T,
UK

Tel: (44) (0) 1932 844526

Email: info@meritpublishing.com
Web: www.meritpublishing.com

merit
PUBLISHING
INTERNATIONAL

About the author

Mario Luca Russo, M.D.

Established in London in the '90s, Mario Luca Russo was born in Venice. He qualified at one of the oldest medical schools in the world, the University of Padua in Italy and subsequently went to work at the famous Great Ormond Street Children's Hospital in London. Dr. Russo worked first as a heart surgeon and later in cosmetic surgery in Naples and in London. But more and more he found himself attracted to non-invasive treatments for protecting and restoring ageing skin, and set up his private practice to pursue this interest.

The Russo Rejuvenation Clinics offer the latest in rejuvenation therapy detailed in this book, from the simplest cosmetic skin-peeling to complex lifting, re-contouring and facial rejuvenation. Only procedures approved to be safe and effective by the US Food and Drugs Administration and by the UK Medical Device Agency are used.

New patients entering one of his clinics first have a private consultation with Dr. Russo and he creates a detailed analysis of their skin, soft tissue and bone structure, so that the program of treatment to be followed is tailored to their individual needs. He also takes digital before and after treatment photos to monitor its success. Dr. Russo is fond of saying that "ageing is optional - with the right skincare from youth and the right treatments as you grow older, you can grow old imperceptibly. Eighty percent of ageing comes down to too much exposure to light," he reminds his patients. Though if harm has been done, there are now highly effective rejuvenation treatments that can redress some of the damage. And since prevention is even better than cure, he has now created his very own skincare range.

In Rome, they used to say 'mens sana in corpore sano' which translates into: 'healthy mind; healthy body', and in that spirit, the Russo Rejuvenation Clinics now also offer Ayurvedic treatments, whose mantra is the re-balancing of body, mind and spirit. These are carried out by therapists from South East Asia.

The Russo Rejuvenation Clinics are in Canada Place Mall, in Canary Warf, East London, and on Devonshire Street in central London. Dr. Russo also has clinics in Milan and Dubai. He continues to lecture at international conferences, including The World Conference of Dermatology.

Contents

Foreword

Most of us have something or other on our skin we would just as soon be without - a mole, scar or a vein. And, of course, everyone eventually gets wrinkles - those tell-tale signs of advancing age. Over the past several years, the removal of these skin imperfections has been made easier by cosmetic lasers and other outpatient procedures. These days, most of my patients have heard quite a bit about these treatments. Unfortunately, much of what they have heard is misleading... lasers are not magic wands; they cannot replace a facelift or produce the flawless complexion of an infant. When used properly, however, lasers and other cosmetic procedures can be used to improve a variety of skin conditions and gently erase the marks of the passing years.

In his book, *Rejuvenating Skin without Surgery*, Dr. Mario Luca Russo provides insight to the processes available to refresh and renew skin on the face and body. Dr. Russo explains a variety of clinical procedures in an easy-to-understand format and the illustrative 'before and after' treatment photos enable readers to visualize the changes that can result from these different processes.

Dr. Russo takes us through the decades of skin life, beginning with the 20s and moving through the 60s and older. Throughout the text, he carefully explains the texture of skin at these milestones and provides detailed discussion regarding appropriate cosmetic procedures to achieve rejuvenation.

For those interested in revitalizing or enhancing their appearances or learning more about the advantages of non-invasive cosmetic procedures, *Rejuvenating Skin without Surgery* is an excellent initiation.

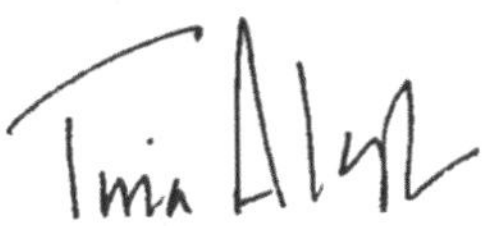

Tina Alster, M.D.
Washington, DC

Dr. Tina Alster founded the Washington Institute of Dermatologic Laser Surgery in Washington, DC in 1990, which was the first independent laser center in the world. She is internationally recognized as an expert clinician, researcher, author and lecturer. Importantly, Dr. Alster has undergone many of the same procedures that she practices, giving her special insight about the clinical experience and outcome.

Introduction

I'd like to tell you about the winding path that has led me to writing this book.

I was born in Venice and trained as a doctor in Padua northern Italy – at the second oldest medical school in the world. I worked first as a heart surgeon in Italy, but I developed an interest in the kind of surgery that corrects heart defects in very young babies and in the early 90s, I came to study at Great Ormond Street, the famous London children's hospital. I had fallen in love with children and the problems they can face early in life. At the time, the first tentative attempts were being made to repair a baby's birth-defects while it was still in its mother's womb – an immensely difficult and delicate task. It is a worthwhile goal because babies with severe birth defects rarely live long after birth, and by operating while they are still sustained within their mothers' bodies you may be able to prolong their lives after they are born.

There is another valuable and unusual thing about operating on babies still in the womb: their wounds heal perfectly, leaving no scar. I became intrigued by this unique characteristic of an un-born baby's skin and wrote my first scientific paper about it. Everybody has noticed the flawless perfection of a baby's skin. The fact that it heals rapidly, with the only slightest scarring, has been known for years. In fact, where skin is concerned it's something of a down-hill journey from birth, or even before. It heals more slowly and less satisfactorily the older you get. And of course it begins to develop blemishes little by little.

What was behind this slow, inevitable decline in skin quality, I wondered? I came to the conclusions that it was caused by light and that as much as 80 percent of it was premature ageing and avoidable. And not just the fierce, hot glare of sunlight from which we are constantly urged to protect ourselves by the liberal use of suntan lotions, but ordinary, cloudy days. Why else can it be that eighty-year-olds can have skin on their buttocks almost as flawless, plump and elastic as that on a baby's bottom? I have seen patients from Japan and the Middle East, where it is fashionable to stay pale, or required by custom to cover the body from top to toe in enveloping clothes, who have skin like a baby's all over their bodies.

This observation led me to my current professional interest in rejuvenation procedures. It became my mission to make people aware of the damage light can do and to offer treatments that corrected it if harm had been done. As a specialist in surgery on children I have practiced reconstructive surgery – the correction of physical deformities or injury. Reconstructive surgery is a marvellous way to correct serious facial defects like a crooked nose or bat-ears. And a facelift, where the surgeon pulls up or takes away skin that has stretched and wrinkled with age and the force of gravity, is indeed a rejuvenating operation – patients may look 10 or more years younger afterwards.

But over the years, I had become more interested in less invasive procedures and above all, in what could be done to prevent skin damage. This is why I have recently developed a medically-formulated, sun-protective skincare range that will reduce the effect of light upon the skin from the start. I discuss this in chapter 7.

In this book, I will show you how you can slow down the ageing process and care for your skin through the decades. As you go through life different treatments will be appropriate. That is why I have taken each decade of life separately, although some treatments are suitable at several different ages. No one should undertake a medical or surgical rejuvenation procedure without understanding fully what can realistically be achieved, what is involved and what risks are entailed. Ultimately, an experienced professional will explain this to you before carrying out any procedure. But I hope this book will make it easier for you to consider what might be right for you and your skin and to assist you in discussing things with an expert. Your skin is an amazing and wonderful organ. Care for it and it will serve you well throughout your life.

Mario Luca Russo, M.D.

CHAPTER 1

Understanding and protecting your skin

What is skin?

Perhaps you are young enough not to have thought much about your skin except to worry about the odd pimple. However old you are it is worth taking a few moments to understand how skin is made and what role it performs for your body so that you may learn to treat it as the uniquely valuable tissue it undoubtedly is.

The skin is the largest organ in your body. It measures as much as two square meters on an adult man and about one and half square meters on the average woman. It's about 70 percent water – which explains why retaining moisture is so important to keep it in good condition.

Think of it this way: your skin, like your eyes and ears, is a doorway to your body. It keeps some things out but lets other things in. The scientific term for this is 'semi permeable' and in fact all the cells of your body, not just skin cells, are surrounded by a fine membrane that carefully regulates what goes in and what gets out. The skin is your first line of defense against potentially harmful things: physical, chemical or bacterial, and it also makes sure you don't lose too much water. Underlying its protective surface are nerves that register things like heat, cold, pressure, pain and pleasure, and send messages to the brain which interprets and reacts to them. The brain acts to correct these sensations if they are nasty (quick; it's cold; put on a sweater) or to prolong them if they are nice (keep stroking the cat's fur). Through the activity of the sweat glands and blood vessels the skin also helps maintain your body at just the right temperature; not too hot; not too cold, whatever goes on outside.

The three layers of skin

The thickness of your skin varies. At its finest, on the eyelids, it is only half a millimeter. On the soles of your feet and palms of your hands it is as much as eight times as thick. Skin may feel smooth, but actually it has an uneven surface and where it is thickest this produces a series of ridges which are the basis of fingerprinting which the police use to track down people who may have been at the scene of a crime. There are three layers: the outer layer known as the epidermis. (Dermis is the Greek word for 'skin' and epi is Greek for 'outer'. You will recognize dermis in lots of words to do with the skin like dermatologist: a doctor who treats skin conditions; and dermabrasion: a rejuvenation technique that removes some of the old, outer layers of skin to reveal fresher, softer layers underneath.) The cells in the epidermis are completely renewed every month. New cells, formed beneath the skin, gradually progress through the layers until they appear in the epidermis, finally to be sloughed off as dead skin cells, or follicles. New cells also form to heal any damage suffered by the skin.

The middle layer of the skin is the dermis, a dense, flexible layer of connective tissue cells and collagen fibers. You will have heard of collagen because this is what gives skin its firmness and resilience in youth but which loses its elasticity as you age. As well as collagen the cells of the dermis contain substances called elastin and hyaluronic acid (HA). The nerves that give you a sense of touch are also located in the dermis.

Underneath the dermis is the deepest layer of the skin, the subcutis (under-skin): a thick cushion of connective tissue, held together by collagen fibers, that contains fat cells and blood vessels and which acts as an energy reservoir, protective padding, and heat insulation all rolled into one. This layer also connects the skin to the various underlying tissue of the body.

Skin changes over time

Imagine you are looking at a grandmother holding her baby grandchild. What are the differences in their skin? The most obvious one is the smoothness of the baby's skin. The underlying bone, muscle and sinew in a baby are all there and working; watch it screw up its face to yell, reach out or kick its legs, but they are almost completely invisible. The layer of fat under the baby's soft, elastic skin – the subcutaneous layer – rounds off all the underlying structures. Now look at the grandma's hands and face. If she has cared for her skin and kept it out of the sun, the skin of her face may still be fair and soft, but it will be covered in small creases and probably pulled into downward folds. On her hands, which have inevitably been exposed to the sun, the bones, blood vessels and sinews will stand out; the knuckles may be enlarged, and there will almost certainly be freckles or the blotches called liver-spots. This is because that subcutaneous fat has all but disappeared, the all-important collagen is no longer bouncy and elastic, and time, the sun, gravity and repeated muscle contractions have taken their toll.

People and faces do not all age at the same rate or in the same way, and the older a person becomes the more noticeable this is. It's easy to tell the age of a child; slightly more difficult when children become adolescents; more difficult still in their 20s and increasingly so through the decades until, by 65, even an experienced health practitioner finds it near impossible to calculate exactly someone's chronological age (their birth date) compared with their physiological age (how they appear) – which may be greater, or less, depending on the genes they have inherited, the care they have taken, and the life they have led. Nevertheless, rapid or gradual, gentle or dramatic, age brings change.

From early youth we peer into the mirror and track the process. In our teens there are the minor blemishes. Only rarely do you see moles or freckles on a baby's skin; these develop only as the skin is exposed to light.

The hormonal changes of adolescence make the skin susceptible to pimples or acne, and maturity also alters the proportions of the face. It becomes longer, particularly between the eyes and mouth, some of the fat padding the cheeks may disappear and bone structure become more apparent.

In the 20s, the effects of muscle contraction begin to create little smile lines round the mouth or at the corners of the eyes plus frown lines between the eyes. This isn't necessarily unattractive but it marks the move from childhood into youth. As faces age a smooth blandness gives way to increased character and individuality.

As time passes, the force of gravity combines with constitutional factors like genes, temperament, reduced hormone and fat-cell production, and behaviors like smoking, poor diet, excess alcohol consumption or sun exposure, to drag the skin into creases. The hands are a real give-away to chronological age because they are almost impossible to keep out of the sun. In addition there is less fat on them to soften the underlying structure than on other parts of the body. On the face, lines and folds become deeper; coloring fades and spots and blotches appear. This is most noticeable in the cheeks, the jaw and the neck, but fine wrinkles also affect the upper and lower eye-lids which can become puffy or hollow, and the lips, which lose plumpness and develop vertical lines round their edges, especially if you smoke. The pupils of the eye dilate less readily and the eyes appear paler.

Things you can do to protect your skin

All this makes depressing reading, nevertheless there is a great deal you yourself can do to protect your skin and slow the effects of ageing, especially if you start young.

A. Your general health

It's not completely true to say 'Look after your health and your skin will look after itself,' but it's not a bad place to start. Good health and contentment shine though your face and general appearance. So start with the basics: eat well and take plenty of exercise and learn how to relax. If you are tired, stressed, eating junk food or drinking too much it will show up in the color, texture and general condition of your skin.

Remember, skin cells are regularly replaced so nutrition is important to maintain them in peak condition.

B. A healthy diet

Whole books are devoted to the healthy diet, and different experts emphasize different things, but broadly speaking it is agreed that you should eat:

- lots of fresh fruit and vegetables
- adequate whole-grain cereals and pulses
- moderate amounts of lean meat, fresh fish (especially oily fish) and eggs

- not too much fat, and as little saturated (bad) fat as possible
- moderate amounts of alcohol – at most a couple of glasses of wine a day
- minimal salt, and as little refined sugar as possible.

The fat story is complicated. Good fats (mono- or unsaturated) are those found in olive oil, nut oils and oily fish, which also includes valuable omega 3 (You hear a lot about this important element in food these days). You probably know about the important role vitamins play in health. Some people choose to take multivitamin pills but if you are eating a balanced, healthy diet you should get all you need from food. You may also have heard about antioxidants. These mysterious, but vital things play a critical role in keeping skin healthy.

Some vitamins are antioxidants: vitamin C, also known as ascorbic acid, found in citrus fruit, peppers, broccoli, Brussels sprouts, kiwi fruit and strawberries, is an antioxidant. So is vitamin E (in nuts, seeds, fish oils, olives, and green leafy vegetables). Vitamin E is particularly important in the diet of the over 65s. Other antioxidants are the minute but important traces of key metals found in food: iron, magnesium, selenium and zinc. This protects against ultraviolet radiation and promotes wound healing so is very important for the skin and probably for healthy eyesight. The body cannot manufacture these micronutrients; they have to come from your diet.

C. A healthy weight

The ideal way to be a healthy weight is to *stay* a steady weight throughout your life. This is easier than you might think if you weigh yourself regularly, but not obsessively, so that you never actually get either much heavier or lighter than is normal for you. There is a great deal of discussion about what weight is healthy and if it really matters to you it is possible to check your weight against standard measurements of body mass; the body mass index (BMI), though this is extremely crude and makes little allowance for build or shape. If you can keep to a stable weight, give or take four or five pounds throughout your adult life and you can be fully active at this weight, then it's probably the right weight for you. There are health problems associated with being either very *over*, or very *under* weight, but there are even more associated with yo-yo dieting and gaining or losing weight rapidly and often, which also leads to stretched skin and wrinkles. Over the age of 65 being slightly overweight, rather than too thin is probably preferable and it will support that youthful subcutaneous layer of fat that plumps-up your skin.

D. Being active

Regular, though not excessive exercise is also more important as you get older. It doesn't have to be playing squash or running. Walking or swimming for 45 minutes, several times a week can be sufficient. If you are concerned to maintain muscle strength and bulk and to keep your joints flexible, then a balanced exercise program, either at home or in the gym, is wise. It should include using all muscle groups including cardiovascular exercise for your heart-muscle, and resistance training, where you lift your own weight (push-ups, sit-ups, squats, and lunges). If you decide to undertake an exercise program, especially if you do it later in life, it's probably sensible to start under expert guidance.

E. Protecting the skin

If you are over 40 you will have noticed the dramatic difference between the skin on your bottom and the skin on your hands. This is because the adult human bottom is only rarely exposed to daylight, unlike the face and hands which are out in the open every day. The harm that can be done to the skin by too much sunlight is well known. Wise people learn to tan little or tan gradually. Sunburn is probably the most damaging, ageing thing that your skin can endure. But few people realize that just being exposed to the atmosphere; the wind, rain and light of any sort, also takes a toll on the skin. No one is suggesting that you cover your skin from top to toe, but protecting the skin, especially the skin of the face and throat from harsh elements, extreme temperatures and ultraviolet light will certainly preserve its youthful appearance for longer.

Another element of do-it-yourself skincare is moisturizing. Moisture loss and fat loss are both things that distinguish older from younger skin. It is the loss of fat cells that makes older skin look thinner and more transparent than young skin. Moisture loss makes it more prone to wrinkle and crack. One important water-retaining and texture-enhancing element in the skin is hyaluronic acid (HA). With age the production of HA is reduced. In addition, the collagen in skin loses its elasticity. HA is present throughout the body but 50 percent of it is located in the middle layer of the skin (the dermis) where it helps keep skin smooth and plump through its remarkable ability to retain up to a thousand times its own weight in water. We will return to HA and collagen when we discuss some of the things professional rejuvenation therapy can do to improve the skin, in addition to those things you can you do for yourself.

F. Moisture inside

You will look after your skin and your body as well, if you drink plenty of fluids every day. If you become dehydrated (short of fluid) it makes it harder for your kidneys to clear waste material from the body. Drink water or fresh fruit juice in preference to strong coffee but tea, especially green tea, is good for you because it contains more of those important antioxidants. Quite how much fluid each person needs each day is a personal thing (Some lose more fluid through perspiration than others).

G. Moisture outside

In addition to internal hydration skin benefits from some external moisturizing. Almost any moisturizer, from the inexpensive to the luxury, expensively-packaged brand, will help, and what you chose is more a matter of personal choice than quality. Moisturizers can contain a number of natural and man-made substances most of which have the ability to combine fat and water as a light emulsion. Some products make strong claims to 'nourish' or 'hydrate' (add water) the skin, but in fact, none of these creams actually penetrates the skin significantly. (If they did – and some medical products do – they would be classed as 'pharmaceuticals' rather than 'cosmetics' and could only be prescribed by doctors, rather than sold freely in supermarkets and department stores). What they actually do is lock in the skin's own moisture and thereby prevent dryness and cracking. The more oil a moisturizer contains, the more effective it is in protecting your skin but the greasier it will feel. Moisturizers in ointment form contain, by definition, 80 percent oil and 20 percent water. Creams, on the other hand, contain 50/50 oil and water, and thus do not provide as effective a barrier against moisture loss as ointments. During the day a light cream that blends into the skin and doesn't leave it feeling sticky usually works best, although richer, greasier ointments are suitable for overnight use.

H. Cleaning the skin

Most beauty advisers will tell you that a good skincare regime has three parts cleanse, tone and moisturize. Only after these three basics should you put on the glamour cosmetics that add color. Again, how you clean your skin is a personal choice. People with dry, delicate skins will probably avoid putting soap or hot water on their faces, but someone with an oily skin may not feel really clean without it. If you wear foundation and other colored cosmetics during the day, a cream or lotion is the most effective cleanser. Toner – usually some kind of mild astringent like Witch-hazel – is a good way of removing excess cleansing lotion, but many people just use cold water. After these two, put on moisturizer or a night-cream.

There is one other skincare product that is a useful tool as your skin becomes older. We explained that skin cells are formed deep down and gradually migrate to the surface where they eventually die and are sloughed off. Dried-out, dead skin cells (follicles) are what make the skin surface look white and powdery, especially when you have been in the sun. On most of your body you can 'exfoliate' (remove dead skin follicles) with a loofah or abrasive-mitt but on the face it is wise to be more cautious and use a special exfoliating cream. This feels a little like rubbing fine sand on your face and should be kept well away from the eyes, but leaves the skin feeling pleasantly smooth and taught, ready for a protective dose of moisturizer.

If you follow these simple rules you should keep your skin in the best condition possible for *your* skin. In chapter 7, I introduce you to my own, scientifically designed skincare range which carries sun protection a step further. Previously it was not possible to protect the skin following cleansing. But new technology makes it possible to devise a cleanser that leaves a fine film of sun-protection-factor (SPF) to guard the skin overnight, and until you apply moisturizer the next day.

CHAPTER 2

Age-check skin in your 20s

"My job involves 'ageing maintenance'. I take care of beautiful women who want to stay beautiful for as long as possible. I only take people on for treatments who already feel good about themselves. I can help to slow the ageing process down, but I can't stop it."

Jean-Louis Sebagh, French Cosmetic Surgeon.

You are in your 20s. You are young and in the prime of life. At twenty, models, swimmers and even tennis players start worrying about being over the hill. Your body achieves its prime in terms of physical strength at a very early age. Fortunately, skill, wisdom and experience make it possible to prolong physical performance.

Your skin is part of your body and you need all your skill and wisdom to protect and preserve the qualities it has in youth when it is in peak condition. From your 20s onward, changes occur that begin to undermine this. At this time your body is still producing a whole new skin for you every month, although the outer layer, made up of dead cells, starts to thicken slightly. If you have been a full time party girl, there may be the suggestion of shadows under your eyes the morning after, and if you have smoked the dreaded cigarettes, the first fine lines may appear around your mouth and eyes.

Your body is no longer running at full steam. It is already beginning to reduce the production of important body chemicals like human growth hormone (HGH), which maintains renewal of skin cells. The quality of the connective tissue and the elastic fibers that help keep the skin supple begin to deteriorate, and as skin cells die off faster than they are replaced the skin starts to look older. In addition, with the passage of time, your skin is inevitably exposed to light.

Eighty percent of premature ageing is caused by exposure, not just to bright sunlight, but to all forms of natural light. Not everyone is able or willing to protect their skin from exposure to light, so even in your 20s you may start to detect signs of damage. If you've managed to avoid sunburn caused by ultraviolet B (UVB) rays, you will have escaped some of the most serious effects of sunlight, but other, more subtle forms of damage occur from exposure to all wavelengths of daylight, indoors and out. The first signs of dyspigmentation – uneven or mottle coloration of the skin and/or small broken veins and skin blemishes, appear at this age.

In addition to its effect on the skin, surface UVA light also penetrates into the middle layer of the skin (the dermis) setting off other changes that tend to show up with ageing. Light can actually damage DNA – the basic building blocks living things are made of – by encouraging the formation of harmful chemicals called oxygen-free radicals. These bad guys can lead to strange, colored blotches on the skin and even to skin cancers if you are unlucky. So the more you protect your skin from exposure to light, at all times of day and all the year round, especially at this early age when the skin is still tender, the better you will preserve its positive, youthful qualities.

With the build-up of dead cells on the surface and the loss of firmness underneath in the middle layer of skin, you can see why the first, fine expression lines begin to appear on the face at this age. These are most likely to turn up in places where there is a lot of movement in the skin; where your facial muscles pull the skin in different directions, such as around the eyes, between the eyes, on the forehead and at the corners of the mouth. With luck, at this stage they will only be visible if you peer in a magnifying mirror in a strong light. The fine lines that form in the skin during your 20s are less than half a micron in depth - that is 0.00002 of a millimeter (1.968503 in.).

The other thing that contributes to these early signs of skin ageing is that the surface layer is beginning to dry out. This is why getting into the habit of a regular, protective skincare routine is vital.

Medical rejuvenation treatments that revitalize the skin in the 20s

Rejuvenation means making young again. Of course, when you are in your 20s your skin is still young – or at least young-*ish*, but taking action before really serious damage has been done makes a lot of sense. There is a range of tried and tested non-surgical medical techniques that may revitalize the youthful appearance of the skin as it begins to show the early signs of ageing.

Microdermabrasion

We have explained that dead skin follicles build-up on the surface of the skin (the epidermis). Most of these are rubbed off naturally against clothing and bedding. But if you remove the powdery outer layer of dead skin cells completely, by light but systematic abrasion (a bit like sanding down paintwork, only gentler) the younger, firmer layer of cells underneath is revealed. This can be done on the face, hands or body and is particularly helpful for the treatment of raised scars, acne scars, black-heads, fine wrinkles, stretch marks and the dark patches or blemishes caused by sun damage. It takes about 20 minutes, is only minimally uncomfortable and requires no anesthetic, so there is no recovery time. You can pop into the clinic during your lunch hour and be back at work in the afternoon with no disruption to your daily routine.

The abrasion is achieved by spraying fine, medical-grade crystals at high velocity onto the skin (a refined version of sandblasting). The crystals are immediately vacuumed away, together with surface layer of dead skin cells. The treatment leaves the skin feeling smooth and taught and looking clearer and fresher. Temporarily it may be slightly reddened because the procedure stimulates the circulation beneath the skin. Best results are achieved with a series of treatments, which gradually reduce imperfections to uncover softer, smoother skin underneath.

There are no complications, and virtually the only people who shouldn't have microdermabrasion, are those who have taken the acne treatment, isotretinion, (Accutane or Roaccutane) at some time in the previous year.

A slightly different form of microdermabrasion is carried out by passing a hand-held wand with abrasive crystals embedded in the tip over the skin and vacuuming away the dead cells dislodged (more like an emery board than sandblasting).

Microdermabrasion is not the same as dermabrasion, which is altogether more radical and virtually obsolete. It has been completely overtaken by the use of lasers and, personally, I wouldn't consider using it.

Chemical skin peels

Microdermabrasion removes the surface layer of dead cells by mechanical action. Skin peels do something similar by applying an active acid solution. It may sound a little frightening until you realize that there is acid in most fruit - apples or oranges - and that this is the sort of solution used for a chemical peel. A range of different naturally occurring or chemical solutions may be used and, depending on which solution and how long it is left on the skin, different thicknesses of skin will peel off exposing younger, smoother skin cells underneath. It is sometimes referred to as 'resurfacing' the skin, although the new surface is not so much applied as uncovered when the old surface is removed. With the old surface go blocked pores, scars and skin blemishes caused by sun damage.

For twenty-year-old skin, only a superficial skin peel is usually recommended. It is a quick and painless treatment that leaves the skin with a healthy glow. The skin is cleansed and the peeling solution applied and left on for about ten minutes, then washed off and neutralized. There may be slight stinging and the skin may momentarily appear pink or even slightly blotchy, like when you have been too close to the fire, but it wears off in a short time and you can go back to your daily routine with no interruption. You can repeat a superficial skin peel after about four or five weeks and some people have one as regularly as they have their hair done.

A medium-depth skin peel removes a bit more of the top layer of skin. The same procedure is followed; cleansing the skin and applying the peel evenly. The solution may stay on longer than for a superficial peel and turn a whitish grey. Cool, saltwater compresses are then applied to neutralize the acid in the peel. The face may swell slightly and the burning sensation may last an hour or more after treatment. With a medium depth peel the skin may take a week to recover completely, or slightly more, depending on how well your skin heals normally. During this period, the skin will feel quite itchy. It first goes brown and then peels, turning bright red, and then finally fades to a fresh pink. It's a little like recovering from sunburn. Medium depth skin peeling is usually not repeated for at least a year.

Deep skin peeling is an altogether more radical treatment and not usually appropriate for the 20-year-old skin. It takes place under local anesthetic and the solution is left on the skin for as long as 30 minutes. It causes blistering rather like sunburn, and is not the sort of procedure you can do in your lunch hour; some patients feel ill afterwards. However, the results are dramatic and can last for as long as 10 years. These days, equally effective treatments may be provided by lasers with fewer side-effects.

The gentlest skin peel solution used for a superficial peel is made from sugar cane and called 'glycolic acid'. It is one of a family of acids used for skin peels known as alpha hydroxyl acids (AHA), of which glycolic is the most active. Others are derived from milk (lactic acid), or unripe fruit (maleic acid). Stronger chemical solutions – salicylic acid, also known at beta hydroxyl acid (BTA) and trichloroacetic acid (TCA) – alone or in combination, are used for deeper skin peels. The strongest solution is phenol, for deep peel only.

After-care

All these rejuvenating skin treatments provide you with a new skin layer which has not previously been exposed to the elements. This means that you must treat it as you would a baby's skin, protecting it from the sun and using only mild, non-irritating cosmetics. A sunscreen is essential and you should avoid the sauna, swimming (in either chlorinated or saltwater), or facials, while the new skins gets used to being exposed to daily activities.

CHAPTER 3
Age-check skin in your 30s

"For men, the big turning points are 40 and 60. For women, they're 30 and 50. For some reason, marriages break up on even decades like 20 and 30 years, not 25 years. I don't know why. But when the men get to 60 they really think that the 30-year-old woman wants them! What a laugh."

Pat Wexler, New York Dermatologist.

Most women grow in confidence and in self-awareness in their 30s. This often has the effect of making them seem more attractive and at ease than they did in early youth. In your 30s you are old enough to know that your body doesn't just take care of itself. It needs a little help from you to keep it in good nick. You will probably have learned how to keep an eye on what you eat and to get out and take some exercise to keep your figure in trim; how to do your hair in a flattering style and hopefully to take good care of your skin. You are already using common sense and know-how to check the ageing process.

It is in their 30s that most people detect the first wrinkles - that is without having to use a magnifying glass and a strong light. This is because the pace at which your skin cells replace themselves is gradually slowing down; the superficial layer of your skin is drying out, and any habitual facial expressions like squinting, smiling or scowling, have encouraged fine lines around eyes, between the brows and at the corners of your mouth. At this stage wrinkles are not a big deal. They are less than 0.5 microns (0.00002 of a millimeter or 1.968503 in.) in depth. But the slowdown of skin cell replacement can make the skin appear duller, and freckles and sunspots begin to become more noticeable. Tiny capillary blood vessels just under the skin surface become slightly enlarged or break leading to little flecks of red or reddened patches on the skin. Basically the skin becomes less even-looking, losing that nice overall smoothness and warmth it had when you were very young.

Beware the heat of the sun

I grew up in Italy where we expect the sun to shine during the summer. Consequently, we take it easy and over several months we gradually build up a tan, which acts to protect the skin against burning and sun damage - because burning is just about the most harmful thing you can do to your skin. This is what I see people do all the time. They go a little crazy when the sun eventually shines; what I call "binge-sunbathing", instead of going out into the sun for a short time each day until they develop a tan.

The younger you are, the more vulnerable your skin and if you get sunburned in youth, you will be at higher risk of skin cancer in your 30s. The most serious form of cancer is malignant melanoma, which is usually blamed on the exposure of tender skin to intense sunlight leading to sunburn and has risen by 40 percent in recent years. The steepest increase has been among men and women in their 30s.

Cancer UK recommends that anyone taking a holiday in the sun should limit sunbathing to before 11am and after 4pm, when the sun is less intense, and cover their skin where exposed with a strong, broad-spectrum sunscreen applied liberally and regularly. In the US, more than 1 million skin cancers are diagnosed each year. That is more than cancers of the prostate, breast, lung, colon, uterus, ovaries, and pancreas combined.

Those who are really passionate about preserving the youthful qualities of their skin may decide they would rather cultivate a 'pale and interesting' look and keep out of the sun altogether, as they do in some Eastern countries. If you decide to wear a self-tanning cream instead of building up a gradual sun tan, remember that these lotions do not offer the same protection - and often no protection - as the real thing.

"The American Cancer Society estimates that about 68,720 new melanomas will be diagnosed in the United States during 2009. Melanoma accounts for less than 5% of skin cancer cases but causes a large majority of skin cancer deaths."

"One theory for why the UK in particular has such high rates of melanoma is that we typically overdo our sun exposure and allow our skin to burn when the weather is good, because for much of the year our climate is bleak."

Nina Goad, British Association of Dermatologists.

Rejuvenation techniques that can restore thirty-year-old skin

Many of the treatments that were suitable for your skin in the 20s are still appropriate when you reach your 30s. Microdermabrasion and mild chemical peels provide a thorough way of exfoliating the dead skin cells from the skin surface and taking with them many of the small blemishes, scars and fine lines that have developed, exposing younger, fresher skin underneath. In addition, laser treatment may be considered appropriate, particularly the laser treatment offered by a Fraxel machine.

Fraxel Laser treatment

The Fraxel Laser performs the same function as microdermabrasion or a chemical skin peel: it removes the surface layer of dead cells together with all the blotches, lines, scars, and wrinkles that have developed, exposing the underlying layer of newer, fresher cells. However, it does this in less time and with fewer side-effects. According to the British Association of Aesthetic Plastic Surgeons (www.baaps.org.uk), it is "possibly more precise and effective."

Other lasers (including the misleadingly named 'Fraxelized Lasers'), if they penetrate all but the most superficial skin layers, are accompanied by the same side-effects as deep skin peels: reddening, swelling, crusting, and peeling, before you get your new skin. But the Fraxel Laser, so-called because it treats only a *fraction* of the skin at one time, doesn't burn because it splits its beam of light into many micro-beams. Each micro-beam penetrates the outer layers of the skin down to the dermis in a fine 'tunnel' called a microthermal treatment zone, leaving a fine network of surrounding skin totally unaffected. In the treatment zones the dermal layer is stimulated to produce new skin cells and collagen which give the skin a plumper and smoother surface. The network of untreated skin in between the treated areas speeds up healing.

Because it is virtually side-effect free you can go ahead and have a second treatment quite soon after the first. The effect is cumulative because each time the network of untreated skin is in a different place. After about three treatments you will have as much as 70 percent new, replacement skin, and with no unpleasant side-effects.

You can fit a Fraxel Laser treatment into a lunch hour easily. It's done under local anesthetic, so the first 45-60 minutes is spent having a relaxing massage while waiting for the anesthetic to take effect. The treatment itself takes up to 30 minutes. There is no discomfort during recovery apart from a slight reddening of the skin, which patients say is rather like having a sunburn that fades in a couple of days.

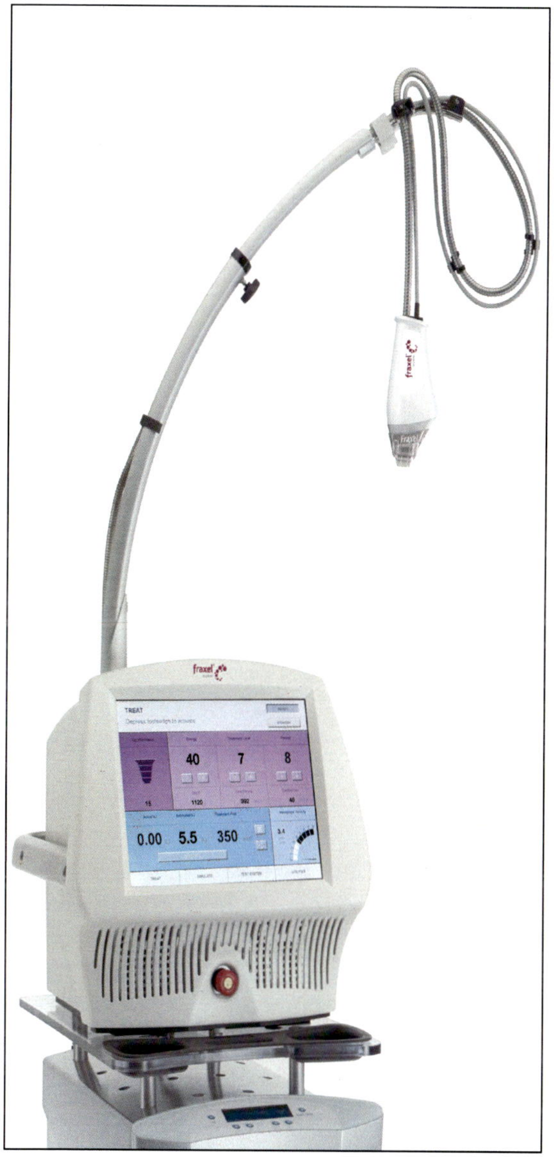

Fraxel re:store™ laser. SOLTA MEDICAL, INC.
Defining a new standard for aesthetic laser skin treatment.

Botox

These days, the trade name Botox is very familiar. It stands for a purified form of the botulinum toxin. If you read up on the science, you could be scared off it completely. The Journal of the American Medical Association calls it; "The most poisonous substance known," and says that a single gram, evenly dispersed, could kill more than one million people. However, the cosmetic form of Botox is nothing like as lethal. It is extremely weak, and the amount we inject just beneath the skin is in minute quantities. It knocks out nerve endings under the skin that control the facial muscles that have been furrowing the forehead, or putting little forked lines between the eyes (known medically as the *gabella furrow*).

"Botox is like grooming now. It's socially acceptable, even expected."

Pat Wexler, New York Dermatologist.

The visual effect is to smooth the wrinkled brow and relax creases. It works best on the upper part of the face: the forehead, between and at the corners of the eyes, but it is also used to soften or erase lines around the mouth or to lift the skin surrounding the eyes by raising the eyebrows, and it can improve the horizontal neck creases that begin to appear in the 30s. Interestingly, botulinum injections are also being used experimentally to provide temporary relief for people with untreatable facial pain.

Botox has been used for cosmetic purposes for more than 20 years. The toxin was identified more than 40 years ago and was first used to cure many different disorders, from cerebral palsy (a serious birth illness that affects muscle control) to excessive sweating. It was also used then for the treatment of squint and blepharospasm (involuntary eyelid spasm). In fact, its potential as a cosmetic treatment was first realized because a patient who had been undergoing treatment for blepharospasm asked to continue treatment after the eye problem had been resolved because of its effects on her wrinkles.

The only people who should avoid having Botox are those who are either pregnant, planning to get pregnant or actually breastfeeding, or those on certain drugs. Before offering you treatment, the doctor at the clinic will certainly check to see whether you are taking any pills. A few people suffer side-effects, the most common being headache, flu-like symptoms, feeling sick, or drooping eyelids. Less frequently, people have also reported redness and swelling at the site of the injection, tingling or pain in the face, disturbed vision and muscle weakness. This last is not surprising since that is what the Botox is intended to do, and sometimes it spreads to muscles it is not designed to affect. Fortunately, these adverse reactions are generally temporary and although these symptoms have been reported in medical trials, they are experienced by very few. The vast majority of Botox injections are free of side-effects.

Having a Botox injection

First, the doctor examines how your face moves when you make certain expressions or movements. This is so that he can judge how the muscles under your face are affecting the skin surface. He will then make a number of small injections of Botox directly into the muscles of your face. No anesthetic is needed and the whole process takes only a few minutes. Any discomfort is usually minimal and brief. It is another of those rejuvenation procedures that you can do in your lunch hour and then continue your normal routine.

The initial effects of Botox become visible within 48 to 72 hours and the maximum effect is reached in one to two weeks. The effect can last up to four months or longer although results vary. But Botox is essentially a temporary treatment. Its affect on your muscles will eventually wear off and you can decide whether or not to have another treatment. Repeated treatment causes some thinning of the muscles, which are injected, and the treatment may last longer using smaller doses of the drug. Long-term trials have not shown any harmful effects of repeated injections on the structure of the muscles treated.

Gabella Furrow Relaxaton (GFX familiarly known as 'No-Tox')

Last year, a more advanced treatment of forehead and the between-the-eyes furrows (gabella) was approved by the US Food and Drug Administration (FDA). Instead of using a toxic chemical, as in Botox, to paralyze the nerves responsible for contracting the skin into wrinkles, GFX knocks them out with a precision pulse of heat, or thermal energy, generated by radio-frequency waves. These are the same radio waves that you pick up with a transistor or cell/mobile phone, but used to produce heat. Heat generated by radio-waves energy is also used in microwave ovens and in surgery as a way of sealing off blood-vessels or killing off cancerous cells. In the case of GFX, the thermal energy is delivered through an insulated bipolar needle inserted near the eyebrows on either side of the forehead. The doctor first delivers a light, stimulating pulse through the needle to ensure it has located the appropriate motor nerve. Then, and once the correct target is isolated, a burst of radiofrequency heat is delivered that knocks out the nerve. The procedure takes about half an hour; results are immediate and the nerve stays non-functional for as long as 18 months - up to four times longer than Botox. And because no product is used, you don't need to do allergy tests first.

Thermage

If GFX can work on the gabella furrow, where else can thermal energy be used? As its name implies, Thermage also uses the heat produced by radiofrequency energy. Thermage is a trade name and other equivalent treatments are dubbed ThermaCool, Aurora, Polaris, and Comet. As with GFX, the amount of heat used in a cosmetic procedure like Thermage is focused and not very strong, and in this instance it is directed, not at nerves that control wrinkles, or upon the skin surfaces, but upon the middle and lower layers of the skin, similar to the way microwaves do. It only indirectly affects the surface skin, tightening it to reduce fine lines and wrinkles. It also helps stimulate the growth of new collagen.

What happens during Thermage?

Thermage should always be carried out by trained operators following a consultation with a doctor. No cuts are made in the skin during treatment and it is effectively painless, although some clinics first apply an anesthetic cream. The operator uses a hand-held piece which contains one or two electrodes. When it touches the skin it delivers the radio-frequency energy to the underlying layers of skin which contains collagen. Some machines include a spray to cool the skin immediately following the action of the radio waves. The treatment may take a few minutes or up to an hour depending on the area of skin to be treated, and no recovery time is needed.

Some machines combine radio-frequency heat with lasers or intense pulsed light, which acts upon uneven pigmentation, fine lines, wrinkles, or surplus hair in the surface layer of skin. Unlike laser treatment, Thermage works just as well on dark or fair skin. A single treatment produces visible improvement, which becomes more noticeable over time and can last for as long as two years. As well as smoothing wrinkles and fine lines, it can improve the contours of the face, tightening the jawline and throat, softening the lines between nose and mouth and on the forehead, and reducing the scarring of acne.

"I use aesthetic procedures to slow down the ageing process. I'm like a picture restorer. I don't want to change the painting; I want to keep your face in good shape for as long as possible by giving back what you're losing. I can't give you back the face you had at 25, but if you come to me two or three times a year at 35 or 40, I can keep your face that way for 20 years without surgery."

Jean-Louis Sebagh,
Parisian Dermatologist.

Side-effects and limitations

Thermage is one of the safest treatments available. With the way it is practiced, it is virtually side-effect and complication free. Occasionally, the skin is left rather red for an hour or two and some people experience some swelling. The treatment is not suitable for people who have pacemakers or any metal implants, as radio-frequency energy may interfere with the way these devices work.

Thermage - Before and After

Thermage uses radio-frequency heat to stimulate the underlying, collagen-containing layers of the skin. It smoothes out wrinkles and fine lines and can also improve the contours of the face. A single treatment produces visible improvement which becomes more noticeable over time and can last for years.

Treatment is effective on various parts of the body. It is particularly successful for the area surrounding the eyes, for the fold connecting the nose and mouth, and even on the backs of arms and the surface of the abdomen.

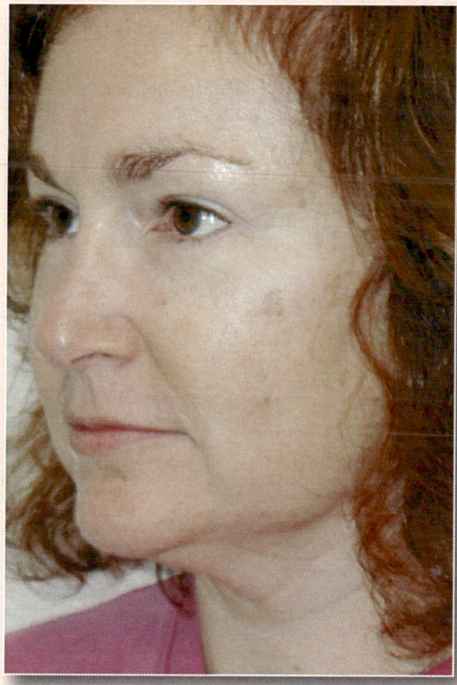

Before Thermage

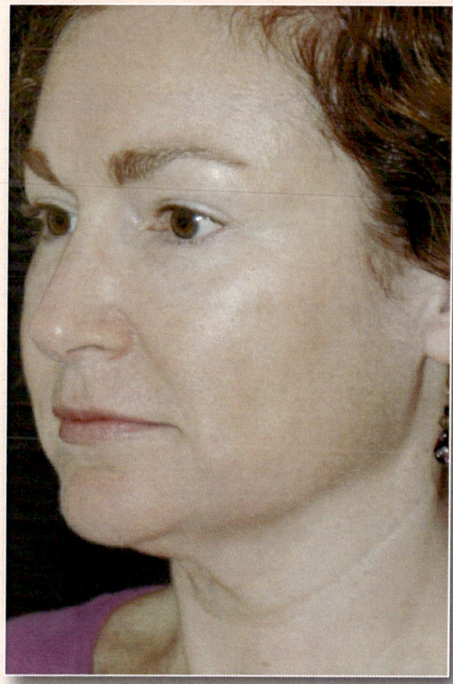

4 Months post treatment

Treatment by Michael Kaminer, M.D.

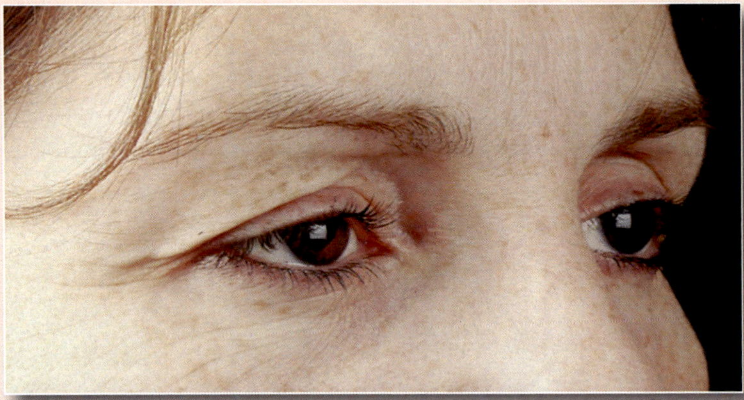

Before Thermage

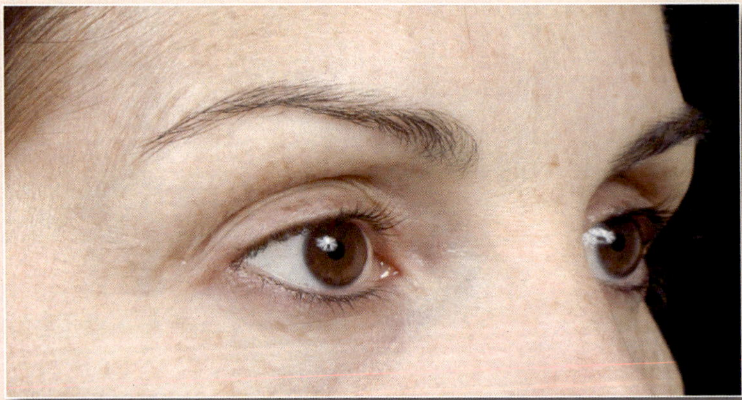

15 Months post treatment

Treatment by Flor Mayoral, M.D.

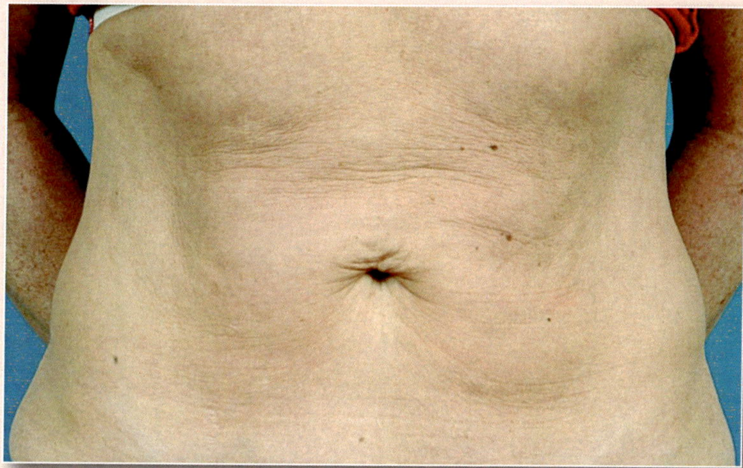

Baseline

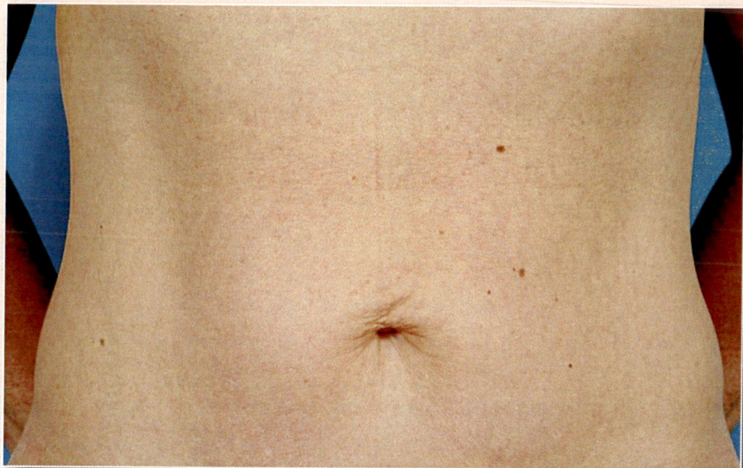

2 Months post treatment

Tummy Treatment Results
Improvement in skin texture, Reduction of wrinkles, Tightening of umbilicus, Overall smoothing and tightening.

Treatment and Photos by Dennis Hammond, M.D., Plastic Surgeon

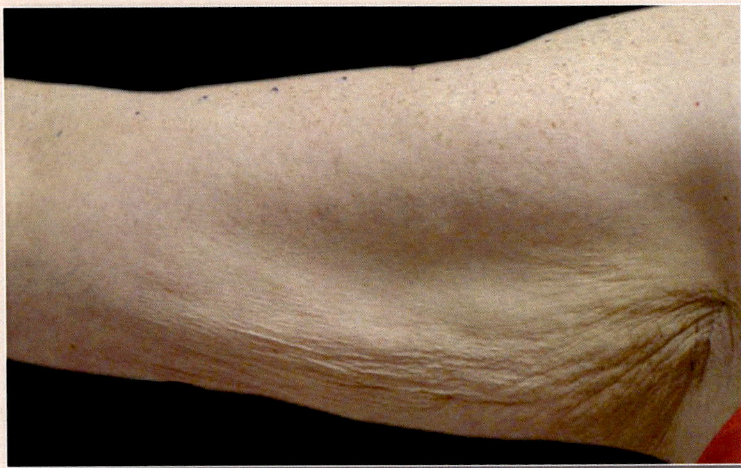

Baseline

Clinical Benefit:
Significant reduction in loose skin and wrinkles, Smoother skin texture and tone, Reduction of crepiness.

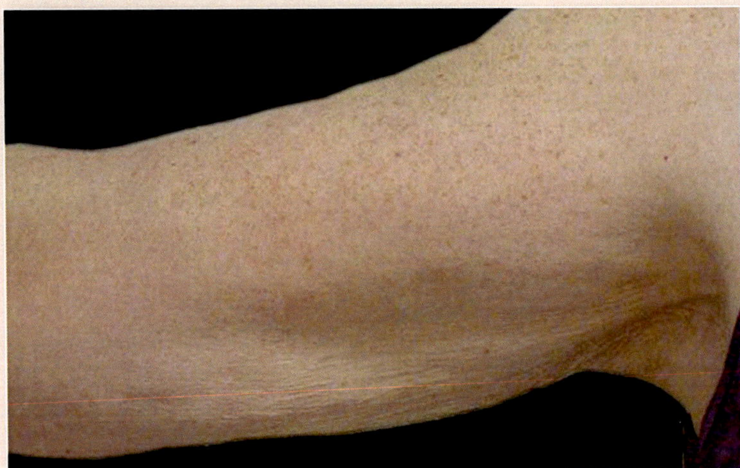

2 Months post treatment

Treatment and Photos by Martin Safko, M.D., Dermatologic Surgeon

Fraxel - Before and After

Fraxel laser treatment removes the surface layer of dead cells together with all the blotches, lines, scars and wrinkles that have developed on it, exposing the underlying layer of newer, fresher cells. Unlike other lasers, it treats only a *fraction* of the skin at one time (hence its name), and it doesn't burn because it splits its beam of light into many microbeams. Each micro-beam penetrates the outer layers of the skin down to the dermis in a fine 'tunnel' leaving a fine network of surrounding skin totally unaffected. The network of untreated skin in between the treated areas speeds up healing.

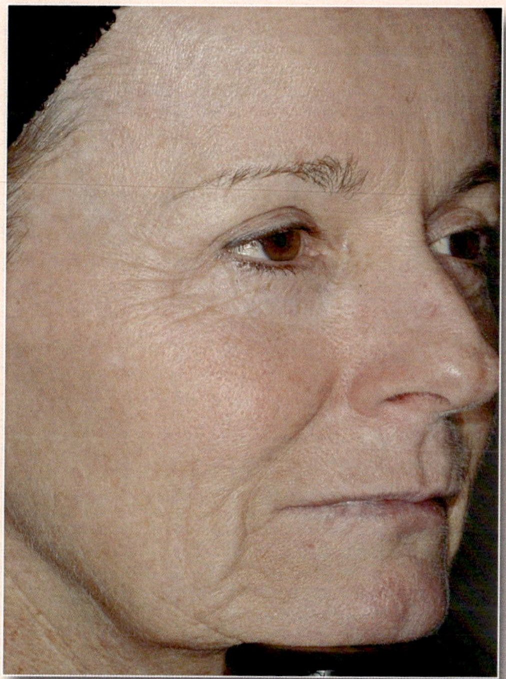

Before Fraxel repair

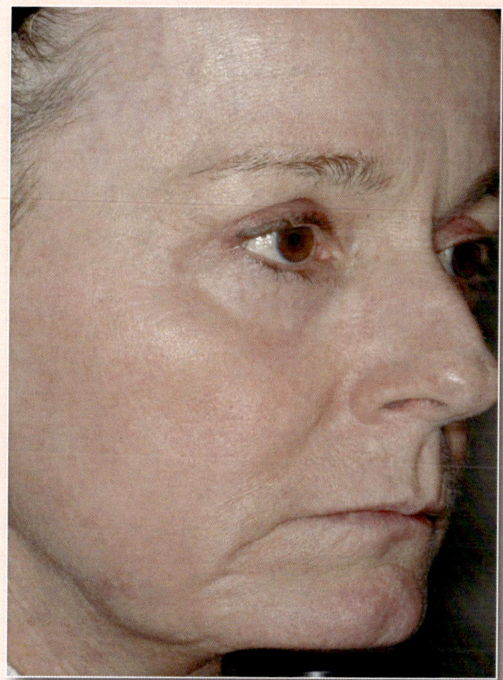

2 Months after 2 treatments

Treatment by C. Zachary, M.D.

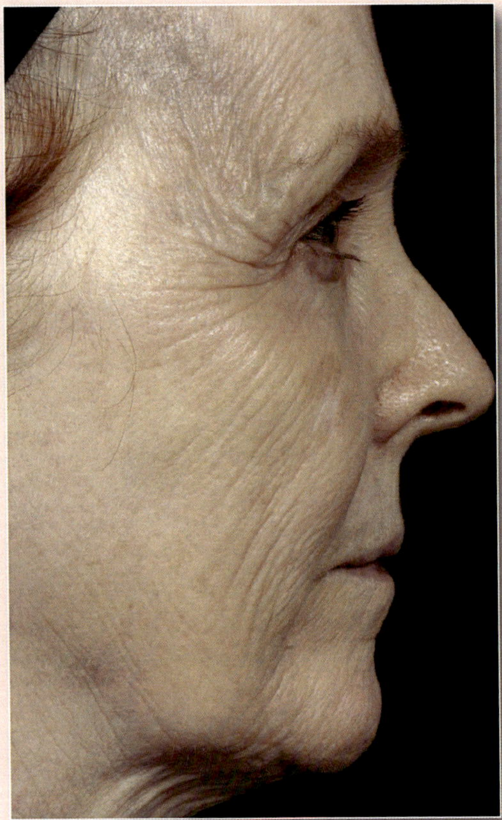

Before Fraxel repair

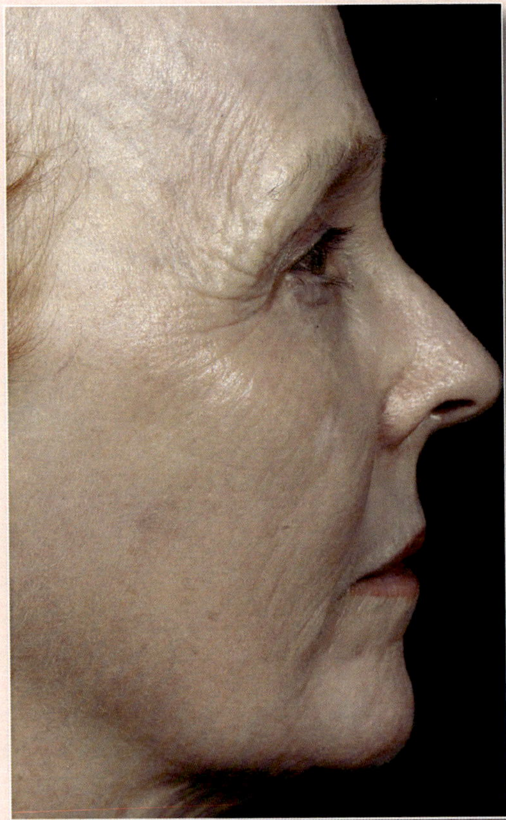

3 Months after 1 treatment

Treatment by Z. Rahman, M.D.

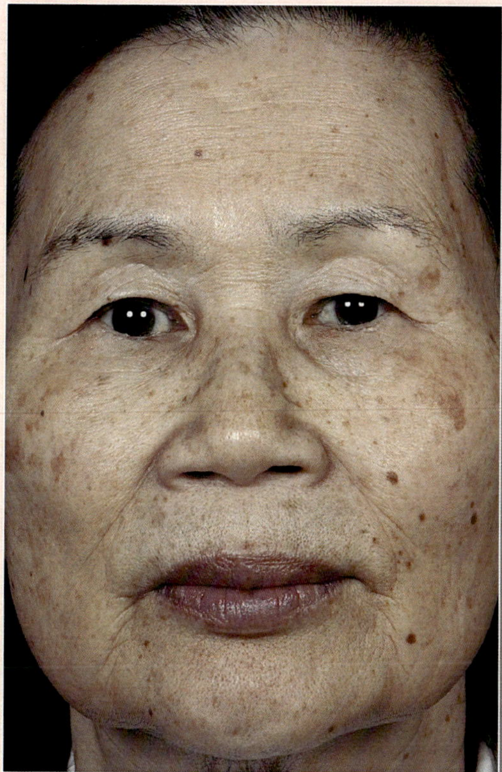

Before Fraxel re:store

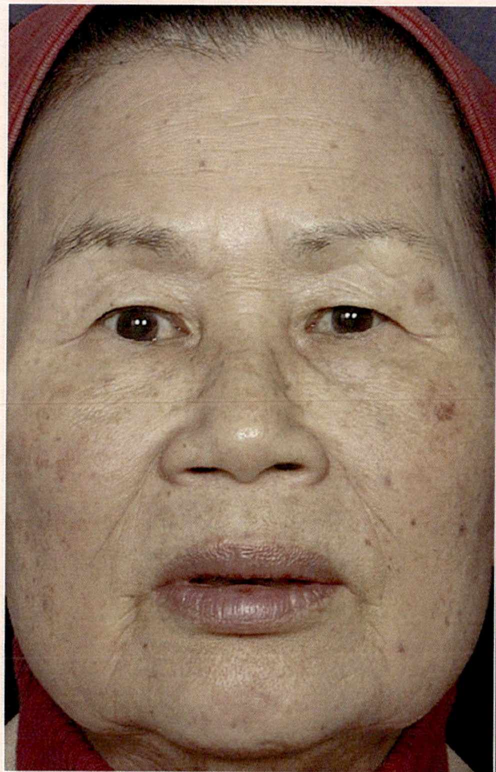

1 Month after 4 treatments

Treatment by G. S. Herron, M.D.

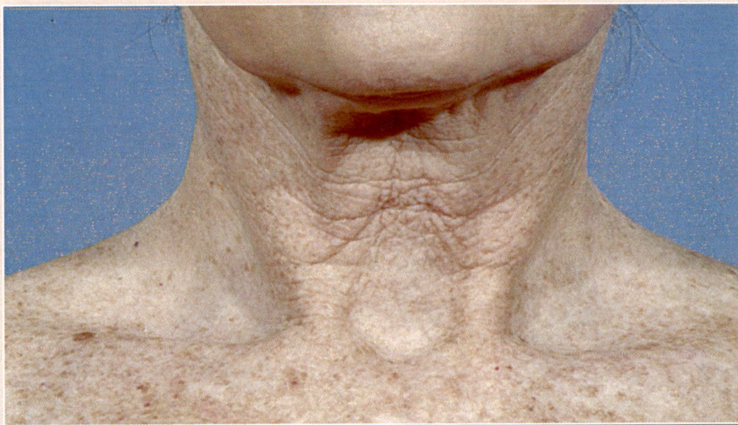

Before Fraxel restore

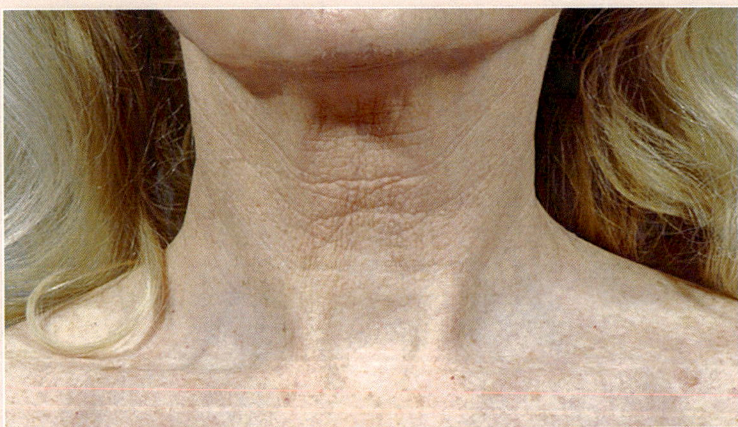

1 Month after 3 treatments

Treatment by J. Burns, M.D.

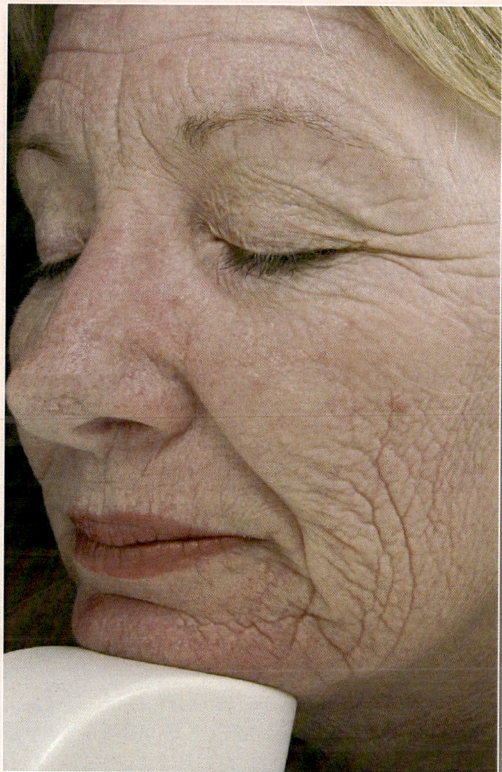

Before Fraxel repair

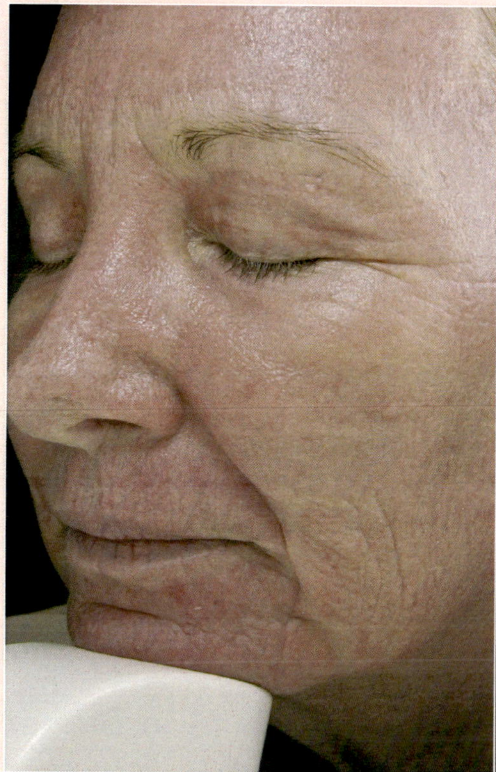

After treatment

Treatment by Steven Weiner, M.D.

CHAPTER 4
Age-check skin in your 40s

"Forty-three is really when you start to look in the mirror and think "Oh my, that's my mother... most of my patients come in miserable at 43."

Pat Wexler, New York Dermatologist.

You are still young in your 40s. If you have taken care of your health and had access to all the benefits of modern life, you have as many years ahead as behind you and more, with luck. If you have a family, it is now hopefully not so demanding and if you have a career, you are probably well established. You have every reason to face life with a smile.

And yet many people hit their 40s riddled with anxiety. At the threshold of middle life, if not middle-age, you ask yourself 'Am I beginning to go downhill?' Socially, mentally and professionally you should be at your peak but physically, you are noticing the tell-tale signs of real ageing. Energy levels not so high? Liver not recovering from a hangover as it did? Do you feel wretched if you don't get your eight hours sleep? And let's face it, your cheeks, throat, breasts, and the backs of your arms are all feeling the pull of gravity, starting the long journey South. Even if you have been really good and kept out of the sun, the wind and other types of weather, that comfortable cushion of fat just under the surface is beginning to thin; the collagen fibers are not so springy. It's time for a really serious age-check.

Forty can be the new 20

It's a cliché we have all heard: 40 is the new 30; 50 the new 40; 60 the new 50 and so on. People, especially women, are keeping their health, vitality and youth longer these days. And with the right care, you too can maintain your skin's youthful appearance without resorting to witchcraft.

Earlier in this book we talked about how to exfoliate the surface layers of dead skin cells in order to expose new, younger cells underneath. These techniques are still useful in your 40s. Whatever your age, a chemical peel uncovers a clearer, blemish-free layer of new skin cells. Botox treatment of the muscles that control facial expression will soften the creases and fine lines caused by scowling, screwing up the eyes or smiling, and fortunately, the more treatments you have had the longer the effects last. Fraxel Laser treatment and

Thermage both covered in chapter 3, continue to play a valuable role in improving the condition and appearance of the skin, and the contours of the face and neck in your 40s. And there are yet more tools in the armory of rejuvenation that you can experiment with.

The complex world of dermal fillers

It's not quite like a crack filler for faces, although dermal (skin) fillers aim to create the same effect - smoothing over the cracks - except that they go *beneath* the skin, not into the cracks. People have experimented with putting various substances into the skin to plump it up, reduce wrinkles and improve the contours of the face since the time of the Pharaohs. Modern fillers were first used in the 19th century when a surgeon experimented with harvesting a patient's own fat and injecting it back under the skin as a cosmetic implant. This kind of filler is called an autologous (patient's own) implant, and various techniques using patients' own fat to enlarge the breasts or make other cosmetic improvements are still in use today. However, their success is limited since the human body is pretty efficient at re-absorbing fat transplanted into the wrong place, so they provide only a temporary boost. When liposuction (vacuuming fat out from under the skin) became fashionable in the late1970s, it gave own-fat implants a new lease of life, and soon after scientists discovered how to filter out the collagen from the harvested fat and process it so that it can be injected somewhere else, although, like all natural products, the body eventually re-absorbs it.

Bad news fillers

In the last century some less satisfactory things were tried as dermal fillers: paraffin for example, which went lumpy after a time, and silicone, which at first was hailed as a wonder implant because it was *inert* – meaning the body didn't either reject it or re-absorb it. But partly *because* the human body didn't react to silicone in the way it does to most foreign bodies by surrounding it with scar tissue, the silicone tended to wander off and turn up, after time, as some bizarre lump or bump in a totally different place from where it had been injected. Eventually, injected silicone was banned, although silicone gel, sealed in a soft plastic bag, is still used for breast implants. These bags are specially designed so that they seal themselves to the chest wall and do *not* turn up behind your back!

In this century, a large number of dermal fillers, man-made or derived from natural substances have been developed. The professional US bodies representing plastic surgeons doing rejuvenation work - also known as *Aesthetic* Surgery (procedures that improve appearance as opposed to correcting damage) - the American Society for Aesthetic Plastic Surgery (ASAPS) and the American Society of Plastic Surgeons (ASPS), reported that in 2007 their members had undertaken more than 1.5 million soft-tissue filler procedures, making dermal fillers the second most popular non-surgical treatment in the US. As advances in technology offered longer lasting fillers, some of the older formulations have dropped in popularity. The newest fillers do not simply 'fill' wrinkles, scars or hollows, they are more ambitious: they aim to restore the *volume* of the fleshy padding covering our bones, recreating its youthful roundness and plumpness.

The ideal filler

The experts all agree that the ideal filler should be *biocompatible* (existing comfortably beside the body's own living tissues), *non-toxic, non-immunogenic*, (neither poisonous nor likely to provoke your body into rejecting it), and *non-migratory* (stays put; doesn't move about like silicone). The dream ticket, which scientists are working on, is a biologically-engineered version of human collagen that could be injected and would then persuade the human body to start producing youthful, springy collagen cells again, just as it did in youth.

Meanwhile, the existing range of dermal fillers vary principally in terms of what is in them and how long they last – from three months to a lifetime. Some also include a local anesthetic to kill the discomfort of the injections. Local anesthetic is generally given before injecting a filler if it is not part of the product. Temporary fillers are re-absorbed, like own-fat implants, though some are engineered to last longer than others. The longest-lasting fillers include natural materials that are compatible with living tissue *plus* another material that is *non-absorbable*. Your might think that permanence is a highly desirable quality in a filler. But in fact, many experts prefer to use something that will eventually be re-absorbed, just in case the patient is dissatisfied with the results, and because faces change with age. What is appropriate at 30 may not be so in 20 years time. The makers of permanent fillers however, claim that they can be safely removed should the patient so wish.

By their trade names you will know them

There are so many names for dermal fillers; some of them so very alike that, like drug names, it can make your head spin. To make life even more complicated, they have different names in different countries. We will try to keep it simple. If you get to the stage of seeking these treatments, your rejuvenation specialist will tell you more about the fillers he/she recommends, or you can find more details on the website given at the end of this section.

Temporary fillers with collagen

You recognize collagen – the cells in the deeper layers of the skin that lose their elasticity and bounce with age. Collagen can be extracted from harvested fat – from either the patient, an animal or from bacteria, and injected to fill out behind lines and wrinkles. The technique was developed more than 30 years ago at Stanford University in California. If animal collagen is used, alone or in combination, a skin test is necessary before treatment to make sure that your body can tolerate the filler. Collagen fillers go under many names, two of which are Zyderm and Zyplast.

Temporary fillers with hyaluronic acid

Perhaps you also remember hyaluronic acid from the first chapter of this book? It is another substance found in the deep layers of the human skin with the important function of holding onto moisture in the skin. Injected beneath wrinkles, hyaluronic acid fillers have a similar plumping effect to collagen fillers, and because it occurs naturally in human skin, you don't have to have a skin test before treatment.

There are versions of both collagen and hyaluronic acid fillers that last a bit longer than others, but all will eventually be re-absorbed by the body. Some doctors use what appears to be extra filler to start with to compensate for the fact that the slight swelling caused by the injection, which adds a temporary plumpness, will subside quite rapidly after treatment. Results usually last between three and six months depending on the individual and also how much has been injected to start with.

Semi-permanent fillers which include non-absorbable 'mini-beads'

Filler can be made to last longer (nine months to a year, or even more) by combining the naturally occurring, but re-absorbable collagen or hyaluronic acid with tiny beads of some material that is *non*-absorbable like silicone. You will come across a lot of long chemical names for these tiny beads, or microspheres, but the only important thing to know about them is that they are inert, like silicone: meaning your body doesn't react to them. This means that after the natural substance, collagen or hyaluronic acid, is absorbed the microspheres stay behind supporting the new plumpness of the skin, and the body's own tissues bind round them to provide a more permanent and long lasting effect. Examples of these longer lasting products include *Artecoll®* and *Radiesse®*.

One filler, Restylane, introduced more than 12 years ago, has led the market in dermal fillers for some years, but recently its pole position has been challenged by Hydrafill and Juvaderm, made by a different company. All products make use of hyaluronic acid from a non-animal source, but, according to Dr Kieren Bong, a rejuvenation specialist working in Glasgow, Scotland, "Hydrafill is the winner" because it contains a higher concentration of hyaluronic acid and makes use of a special process that mimics the way the cells bond to one-another in normal skin called cross-linking.

This makes for a particularly smooth gel that flows easily into the skin. This easy flow also means that the filler looks even more natural and there is less bruising as a side-effect of the treatment, according to Dr Bong. The cross-linking also makes it longer-lasting, typically six to nine months, compared with Resylane's three to six. Among its added attractions, Hydrafill is also approved for every kind of skin tone, including black or Asian skins.

Other long-lasting fillers

A slightly different approach to fillers comes from a French company, which makes *Sculptra™*. These man-made fillers contain materials that are broken down by the body over a period of months, but before this happens they persuade the body to grow new collagen cells. Results can last to up to three years or more. The effects of *Sculptra* take four to five weeks to appear while the body reacts to the filler.

Treatment with dermal fillers

Ideally, dermal fillers should be injected by a trained doctor. A skin test to make sure you don't have an allergic reaction will be necessary if the product includes an animal-derived collagen or hyaluronic acid (less common these days). Treatment can take from 30 minutes to an hour, depending chiefly on how large an area is being treated. A local anesthetic may be included with the filler or applied in advance to prevent discomfort. The clinic may put an ice pack on the site of the injection before and after to reduce swelling and bleeding if you have had a large area of skin treated, or if you bleed easily, you may be advised not to take aspirin for any pain because this drug encourages bleeding. Recovery time depends on the individual patient, on how much filler has been injected, and what kind. The skin may be rather red and bruised for a few hours or a few days. The risk of infection following dermal fillers is low, although anyone who had suffered from cold sores may be advised to take an antiviral medicine like Zovirex that will head this risk off while healing takes place.

"I love fillers… It's all about having those convex surfaces to reflect light."

Frederic Brandt, New York Dermatologist to Observer Woman.

The market for dermal fillers is estimated to be worth millions and appears to be growing as new products are approved and come on to the market every year. It can be a confusing marketplace, and for a wealth of well-informed, no-hype information if you want to know more about dermal fillers before actually consulting a clinic, we recommend the website: www.consultingroom.com. Some dermatologists swear by fillers because they restore volume to faces that have lost their fatty padding as they age, unlike cosmetic surgery (see the next chapter), which only takes away the skin that has become loose or wrinkled without its sub-structure. Other dermatologists are more reserved about them since it is easy to overdo filler and end up with an unnatural, characterless look.

Speaking personally, I have to admit that I do not like fillers. I don't think they address the real cause of the problem. They are often used to fill the nasal-labial fold (the one that develops from the corner of the nose to the side of the mouth), but I think it looks unnatural and there is always the risk that in the soft tissue of the face the filler will migrate to some unintended location. The only place where I am happy using fillers is to correct the shape of the nose, or for the lips, where it is possible to inject the filler from *inside* the mouth for a softer effect. I think you get a much better effect with Fraxel Lasers, which really repair the skin and enable it to retain more moisture, rather than be remodeled with fillers.

Cosmetic surgery

In the US, non-surgical cosmetic treatments, such as peels, lasers, Botox, liposuction and fillers, have increased by an amazing 754 percent since 1997 compared with only 114 percent for cosmetic surgery. Nevertheless, there are things that can only be done with the knife and people first start to consider this more radical rejuvenation treatment in their 40s and 50s. It is a large subject area and we have put it into a separate chapter.

CHAPTER 5
Cosmetic surgery for the 40s and 50s

"Life-expectancy in developed countries is increasing year by year: it used to be 70, now it's more than 80 (for a woman); any minute it will be in the 90s. You can't try to look 30 indefinitely. You're going to have to change the way you look. As we enter our 90s, we don't want to walk around looking like the Dannon yogurt lady."

Pat Wexler, New York Dermatologist.

Your 40s or more particularly, your 50s are decades when you reassess your life. You are no longer living in the fast lane: the tempo has eased; the beat is less insistent. Less hectic, hopefully calmer waters are ahead of you. But it is a period when it becomes even more important to take care of your health and appearance.

Getting older is very much a matter of everything slowing down – the rate at which your skin cells replace themselves, the rate at which your liver cleans out toxins like alcohol, and the amount of important hormones, like estrogen, which your body makes. Estrogen is one of the hormones that regulates fertility in women, and at some time between 45 and 55 all this changes and women face the 'change of life'- the menopause - so-called because the monthly periods (menses) stop. But there is more to the menopause than simply not having any more periods, which many women greet with relief. Hormones like estrogen have an effect on all sorts of things other than the monthly cycle of making eggs and discarding them if you don't get pregnant. They affect your skin, your bones, your hair, your sleep pattern, your sex drive, and your energy levels.

Looking after your health during the menopause requires a book all to itself. Here, we can only deal with what happens to your outward appearance. And at this time of life, cosmetic surgery can restore your confidence and give you a lift in more ways than one.

Everything heading South

Thinking about having cosmetic surgery does not mean you should throw the rest of your beauty routine to the winds. Basic skin care is never more important than now, because your skin is getting drier; shedding dead cells more slowly; areas of uneven color - not just dark blotches and freckles, but little white patches - start to appear on the skin where it has been exposed to sunlight, and that all important fatty layer beneath the skin has grown thin and lacking in spongy bounce. Where the skin is no longer stretched taut it begins to sag downwards because it has lost its elasticity. Chemical peels and Fraxel treatments will help combat the uneven color tones and expose newer, fresher layers of skin. Thermage and dermal fillers will fill out some of the lines and creases, and Botox will relax the muscles that are drawing them tighter. But when it comes to combating the downward drag of gravity, nothing beats surgery.

Cosmetic surgery is not only used to combat ageing, of course. Younger people have it to correct disfiguring physical traits like a hooked nose, bat-ears, or to remold other features that are conspicuous or which make them feel self-conscious. But cosmetic surgery is particularly successful at removing stretched, wrinkly skin that can spoil the contour of neck, jaw and eyes in your 40s and 50s, and restoring some of the clean lines the face had when younger. 'It's a little like ironing your skin,' said one satisfied customer; although cosmetic surgeons do not just smooth out wrinkles, they actually cut away the excess skin that hangs around contributing to them.

Which cosmetic procedure is right for you? People's faces do not all age in the same way. Some may wish to treat a wrinkly neck, or the beginnings of those hang-dog jowls either side of their mouth. Others worry about creases forming round the eyes. You may decide to try one operation or more. The cosmetic surgeon will give you advice, but ultimately it's up to you.

Eyelid lift

The medical name for surgery to the eyelids is blepharoplasty. The first bit of the word means eyelid and the 'plasty' means to change the shape. It's one of the most popular and successful cosmetic surgical procedures. Eyelid surgery can remove drooping upper lids or reduce bags underneath or both together, and it can be combined with surgery to other parts of the face. Large, deep-set eyes are sometimes the first to show those tell-tale signs of ageing, and removing the excess skin, with perhaps some of the underlying fat or muscle, revives their appearance dramatically.

For the upper eyelid, the surgeon makes a cut in the natural crease line between actual lid and the skin stretching over the brow, about a centimeter, or quarter of an inch, above the eyelashes. If there are deep crows' feet at the corner of the eye, the cutting line can be extended outwards - like drawing a line with an eye pencil. The surgeon then carefully separates the skin from the layers underneath, removes any excess fat, and trims the sagging muscle and skin so that the cut can be closed up again with fine stitches or adhesive tabs.

For the lower eyelid, the line of the cut runs closely under the eyelashes – again, rather like the make-up on an Egyptian Pharaoh, and the skin is then separated from the underlying layers and lifted gently up and out until all folds or wrinkles are smoothed out and then surplus skin is then trimmed off. The line of the cut is sealed with fine stitches or adhesive tabs. You can see why it is called a 'tuck'. In fact, the techniques of face lifting are like tailoring in more ways than one.

The operation takes just over three hours. It is usually done under general anesthetic so an overnight stay in hospital is necessary. An upper eyelid lift alone can be done as day surgery. By the time the patient awakens from the anesthetic, there is no real pain, although he or she feels a little bruised and sore and there may initially be some swelling. The eyelids may feel a little dry at first and the surgeon will probably offer you eye drops or a lubricating cream. If stitches have been used to close the incision, they are usually taken out after about five days. The bruising takes a bit longer to clear, and runs through all the colors of the rainbow, so hang onto your shades for a couple of weeks.

The amount of scarring varies between individuals and according to your skin-type, but the line of the scars follow the natural contour of the eye and is deliberately made where most women apply make-up, so they are not very noticeable once healed. Recovery time also varies from person to person. Some people are back into their routine within a week; others take two or three weeks out. Most people are delighted with the results because it really does return the eyes to the clearer, less tired appearance they had 10 years ago. And cosmetic surgery, unlike many other rejuvenating procedures, is permanent. You will continue to age, but from the vantage point that the surgery has returned you to.

A short-scar or mini-facelift

This is the least radical of facelifts and the most suited to someone in their 40s or 50s when the signs of ageing are not yet severe. In a short-scar lift, surgeons make an incision in the skin and remove some of the excess tissue, just as they do for an eyelid lift. The difference between short-scar, or mini, and a full facelift is chiefly in the size of the scar left behind after the operation and the quantity of tissue that is removed during the procedure, though these differences also mean the operation differs in other ways too.

You can see for yourself what a facelift can achieve if you take your two hands and use them to pull back and up the loose skin around your face and neck. If a very gentle movement - index finger to your temples and pushing back your ears - makes you look 10 years younger, you may only need a short-scar lift. If you need to spread your fingers to behind your ears and push, not only your temples and ear lobes but the skin of the neck by pushing up your scalp behind your ears, the pull of gravity has really been working and you may need a full facelift (see the next chapter).

Where and what scars

People are often concerned about scarring when thinking about having a facelift but in practice these are nothing to write home about. How noticeable scars are depends partly on skin type, but also on things like smoking. The vast majority of cosmetic surgeons won't touch you unless you give up smoking before they operate because smoking really hinders healing. But given good health behavior and the average skin type, the scars that remain after a facelift are minimal. This is because they are mostly either on or behind the hair line, so that hair grows back and covers them. A really tiny scar sometimes results from an incision made in front of the ear – no more than an inch. But as this is at the boundary of the ear itself it is virtually invisible once healing has taken place. The exact position of incisions, hence scars, depends on the shape of your face and the growth of your hair.

In a short-scar or mini-facelift, surgeons can usually achieve enough tightening of the skin by cutting only on the temples, along or behind the hairline, and possibly in front of the ear down to the earlobe, or occasionally inside the ear, and then pulling the skin taught and cutting off the surplus tissue before securing the skin in its new position. The operation is usually done under a general anesthetic involving one night in a hospital, though some surgeons do the procedure called a 'twilight' with local a anesthetic and strong dose of a sedative, so that the patient falls into a deep sleep, feeling and remembering very little.

There is some bleeding, of course, while you are asleep, so that to begin with there will be dressings on the stitches, but these do not have to stay in place for long. Any stitches that have been used are usually removed about five days later. There will be slight swelling and quite a lot of bruising that clears slowly, running through a kaleidoscope of colors, but you will feel quite normal in yourself after a few days. People vary, but the bruising has usually disappeared by three weeks. With careful camouflage, you can get back into your routine before this.

A mini-facelift can be combined with liposuction, which is the removal of surplus fat by suction, if the jaw has become 'jowly', or with an eyelid lift, or with dermal filler for those small pursed creases round the edge of the lips. The effects are highly satisfying for the person having the treatment but most of your friends and relations will probably just say, "You look really well!"

You will, of course, continue to grow older and gravity doesn't get any weaker over the years, but after a facelift your appearance goes back 10 years or more and you start ageing from that point.

The cost of cosmetic surgery is like a piece of string – it can vary widely – chiefly in relation to where it is carried out (big cities are more expensive). You should bear in mind that with cosmetic surgery you will also have to pay, not just for your surgeon, but for the services of an anesthetist as well, plus a stay in a private clinic for a night or two.

CHAPTER 6
Age-check your skin in your 60s and 70s

"A 60-year-old now thinks differently from how a 60-year-old did 10 years ago and certainly 20 years ago. I think the changes we've seen in the cosmetic industry are very much driven by the ageing baby-boomer population. You now get people who are going into second careers and want to look good. Even people going into retirement want to look good."

Dr Tina Alster, Director of The Washington Institute of Dermatologic Laser Surgery.

There are vital, fascinating, and fabulous looking women aged 60 to 80, and don't you forget it. Think Helen Mirren; think Sophia Loren; think Elizabeth Taylor. There are distinguished looking men, too, such as Sidney Poitier, Bill Clinton and Clint Eastwood. Not only are many 60, 70, 80 year olds still in fine fettle, many continue to fill positions of power and influence. Maybe at this age, as 80-year-old and still twinkling writer Katherine Whitehorn puts it, "You are unlikely to charm anyone at a party with the melting invitation of your smile" but then by this age you are less preoccupied with inviting people at parties and more concerned with getting home to bed in time, walking the dog or planning where you are next going to travel.

Although no amount of conscientious skincare or cosmetic surgery can now make you look 20, this period in your life fortunately coincides with changing priorities. You probably don't want to look 20 again, let alone *be* 20 - an age when many of us were totally confused. But you do want to hold onto whatever good looks and good health you already have.

The older people become, the more difficult it is to judge age by appearance. Whereas an expert examining a child of 10, an adolescent of 16 or a young woman of 25 can be pretty confident of their biological age, by the time we reach 60, the year when we were born is much harder to guess by physical appearance alone, because we do not all age at the same rate. We have all seen people who look middle aged at 35 as well as blooming 60-year-olds going on 40. The genes you inherit obviously play a part in this, but so does the life you lead. A happy, healthy, sheltered life will preserves the body more than one wracked by misfortune, unhappiness and outdoor labor. So if you've managed to look after your body so far, don't give up now.

Skin care for the 60s and 70s

Caring for the skin becomes increasingly important as you grow older. Your body produces less of the natural oils that keep the skin moist, and in addition, the skin becomes less efficient at holding onto moisture. You need to moisturize not only your face and neck and hands, but your legs, feet, throat, arms - especially the elbows - and shoulders; in fact all those parts of your body that have been exposed to the atmosphere for 60 years. The routine of cleanse, moisturize, nourish is something that should become as instinctive as cleaning your teeth at night, and you should do it whenever you shower or bathe.

Purely cosmetic products on the other hand become slightly less important. Yes, you still need some color on your mouth and cheeks - inevitably, since you have less natural color there now - and a little definition on your eyes and eye-lashes, especially if you are fair and blue-eyed and your features seem to be disappearing into your face. And you can still put on the full amount for special occasions, probably at night. But by day you should apply cosmetics with a light touch. Too much make-up, foundation, powder, as well as lipstick, eye-shadow, and rouge, actually emphasizes creased skin, enlarged pores and blunted contours. Apply these with increasing subtlety as you grow older. Dated make-up, like a dated hairstyle, betrays your age quicker than the pop music you enjoy or the slang you use.

Skin treatments for the 60s and 70s

Some rejuvenations treatments are less suitable for a 60-70 year-old skin. The skin has become much thinner and more transparent. The bones and blood vessels under the skin show up because the fatty layer of padding underneath has all but disappeared. Dermabrasion and chemical peels are not usually suitable for this sort of skin. Skin coloration becomes increasingly uneven at this age - not only freckles and brown blotches (liver spots), but little white flecks where the cells that used to color the skin have given up completely. This unevenness can still be improved with Fraxel treatment or Thermage, and the underlying layers of the skin will be encouraged to produce new cells. Dermal fillers may still be used, although with increasing caution because as the skin surface becomes more thin and fragile, any unevenness underneath will show through.

Carbon dioxide (CO2) and erbium laser skin resurfacing

"A blast of carbon dioxide could be better at erasing wrinkles than face creams," said the headline in London's *Daily Mail* in July 2008. Carbon dioxide resurfacing is, in fact, another form of laser surgery which was offered as a rejuvenation treatment more than 20 years ago. However, it fell out of fashion because many patients suffered unacceptable side-effects, such as discoloration of the skin and scarring.

The new excitement in the press was caused by a report in a serious medical journal: *Archives of Facial Plastic Surgery*, on research carried out at the University of Michigan. The study was of only 47 patients, but the team claimed significant results: "...up to 50 percent fewer lines and wrinkles", after a period of two and a half years, although nearly half the study group still had some side-effects.

The problem with research on a very small number of people is that you have no idea how a larger group of people might be affected. The side-effects picked up in a small study might emerge as more common, or they might be rarer; the good results less frequent or, of course, more frequent. Carbon dioxide resurfacing works by heating the skin so that the tiny molecules of water in and around it are turned into steam. This stimulates the body to produce collagen to repair the damage – rather as it does in response to the tiny beads injected with dermal fillers. But even in this latest, well-received study, quite a few patients suffered side-effects of skin discoloration or acne, and the discoloration was still apparent two years later.

The erbium laser is less invasive than CO2 resurfacing. It also heats the molecules of water in the skin to remove superficial lines to moderately deep wrinkles together with the outer layers of the skin, but the layers removed are finer and there is less discomfort and fewer side-effects, and a more rapid recovery than with CO2 resurfacing. But it can still produce dramatic results. It also activates collagen which may further tighten the skin. Bandaging is sometimes necessary for a few days afterward, as it is for CO2 resurfacing, and after a week ointment is applied to prevent the slight risk of scarring, but in seven to 10 days, you will be able to resume normal activities.

Facelifts in your 60s and 70s

In an earlier chapter we discussed forms of cosmetic surgery that lift and remove skin from the face and neck when non-invasive skin treatments are insufficient to reverse all the signs of ageing. If you have had one of these minor lifts - a mini or short-scar facelift, in your 40s or 50s, after 10 or 15 years you may still find the wrinkles and hollows are starting to be noticeable again. A second mini-lift could then be recommended. However, if you avoided surgery when younger but decide to try it for the first time in your 60s or even 70s, you will probably need something a little more radical than one of the mini-lifts: a full facelift.

What does the surgeon do while I am asleep?

A full facelift involves removing excess, loose skin from the face and neck and securing the remaining tightened skin firmly to the scalp behind the hairline, all while the patient is asleep under general anesthetic. You can get some idea of the effect of a facelift by using your fingertips to push the skin up on either side of your face. Spread the fingers from your temples to behind your ears and push gently, not too tight, and you will see the wrinkles disappear. The cutting line starts where you put your little fingers: high on the temples inside the hair-line. Push here and you will see that this pulls the skin around the eyes and on the brow tighter, removing creases and wrinkles - it's almost like ironing your face. Occasionally, if the folds of skin round the eyes are too heavy to pull up from the side it may be necessary to make a cut above and below the eye, behind the eye-lashes and remove this loose skin separately (See Eyelid lift in the previous chapter).

The facelift cutting line continues down in the slight groove in front of the ear, under the earlobe and then tracks back into the hairline on the bony promontory just behind the ear. Some surgeons, having cut the skin then carefully separate it from the underlying tissues. They can then gently lift it up and out, remodeling it over the underlying structure, before cutting off the surplus skin and a securing it with stitches or clips to the scalp. Some surgeons take away some of the underlying tissue as well as skin. It all depends on the individual face and how it has changed with age. Occasionally, it is necessary to add an extra cut under the chin to remove skin or fatty tissue blunting the jawline. This cutting line is also well disguised.

A facelift takes from two to three hours. Patients are sometimes asked to go into a hospital or clinic the night before to be prepared for surgery. They then stay a night afterward so that the doctors can check that they have fully recovered from the operation. Any bandaging is removed before you go home. Stitches are removed about five days later. If metal clips have been used to secure the new skin line, these usually stay in place for up to two weeks. There is inevitably quite a bit of bruising, which starts on the face (sunglasses and headscarf might be advised) and gradually fades down the throat. Some patients have a bit of swelling to begin with and doctors will advise you to sleep with your head up on a pile of pillows to discourage this.

Vigorous exercise is also discouraged for a week or two, but otherwise there is no reason why you shouldn't go back to work or take up your normal everyday life as soon as you are confident no one is going to ask who gave you the black eyes, The scaring around your ears or in your hairline gradually fades over three to six months. The surgeon usually asks to see you after about six months to check that everything has healed well and to judge the results.

Healing and scarring vary from patient to patient. The surgeon will certainly tell you not to smoke before the surgery or immediately after the operation because smoking slows down the healing process. If you can use the break to give it up for good, better still. Most people who have had a facelift feel really pleased with the results. It's like renewing your acquaintance with the face you used to see in the mirror 10 years ago. You will, of course, continue to age but it will start from 10 years earlier.

"You can make someone's face look like a 20-year-old's, pretty close. Neck and chest and hands are harder. If you see someone with a face that doesn't match their neck, chest and hands, you know they have had work done. They still look old."

Dr Tina Alster, Director of The Washington Institute of Dermatologic Laser Surgery.

One word of warning before you have a facelift: your face may look 10 years younger, but remember, the rest of you - hands, arms, knees - stays the same age.

Cosmetic work on your teeth

Cosmetic dentistry is sometimes referred to as 'a smile makeover'. Apparently more than 75 percent of people are not confident enough to smile for a photograph.

We don't usually think of it in terms of rejuvenation, but cleaning, polishing, veneering, capping, bridging, and many forms of standard dentistry are in fact a way of turning back the clock and making your teeth, not just healthier, but younger or younger looking. If you are having the wrinkles ironed out of your face there is something to be said for enhancing the brilliance of your smile.

People's teeth are not all the same color to start with. Some are whiter than others; some yellowish or grey-toned. As you grow older so does your tooth enamel. It gets scratched and worn and hence picks up stains more easily. This can be aggravated by lifestyle and diet. Superficial stains can be removed by brushing with a tooth-whitening toothpaste and a periodic scale and polish with a professional hygienist. Resistant stains may respond to a prophyflex removal treatment. This is a powerful jet of compressed air, water and fine, mildly-abrasive particles fired at the tooth surface under high pressure; a dental version of sandblasting or microdermabrasion of the skin. Deeply embedded stains that have worked their way into the structure of the teeth, such as black coffee, red wine, curry, or nicotine stains from smoking, sometimes resist even this treatment and may require whitening carried out by a dentist using peroxide that penetrates the tooth surface and bleaches the enamel.

Some stains defy even professional tooth whitening, in which case the next stage is to apply a veneer. A veneer is a wafer-thin skin or shell of tooth-colored material which is cemented to the front of the tooth rather like an artificial fingernail. The added attraction of fitting a veneer is that, you not only have a new, undamaged surface to your tooth but the dentist can correct any gaps, crookedness or unevenness of your teeth. You can see a demonstration of how this is carried out on a cosmetic dentistry website: (http://www.cosmeticdentistryguide.co.uk/veneers.html). These are not high cost procedures and really do give your smile a lift.

Dental implants

The previous generation of 60 to 70 year-olds often had a plate or a full set of false teeth by the time they reached this age. These days, free dentistry for children and the use of dental fluoride - in toothpaste or in the water supply - has produced adults with much healthier teeth, although poor diet will still undermine the best dentistry in the world. In addition, there is improved understanding of how to treat gum disease. This is more common in middle age because the gums shrink, leaving the area around the tooth border exposed and prone to infection and decay.

In the past, dentists often pulled out teeth loosened by gum disease; these days they encourage conservation by teaching thorough brushing and flossing, and most of us reach old age with a near full set of our own teeth. However, in some cases if your teeth have had so many filings they are crumbling away, the dentist may recommend crowns or implants, made of titanium. These are so natural you tend to forget you have them, and they are infinitely preferable to the old-fashioned plate with false teeth attached. Dental implants are sometimes referred to as your 'third set' of teeth, following your baby teeth and your adult teeth. You can see this explained well at the same website: http://www.cosmeticdentistryguide.co.uk/implants.html.

CHAPTER 7
Skincare designed by dermatologists

Thank goodness for rejuvenation treatments. They are improving every year. Nevertheless, the ideal treatment is one that prevents skin damage in the first place.

In fact, the ideal skincare regime is very simple. We touched upon it in the very first chapter of this book: *Understanding and caring for your skin*. You clean your skin daily - exactly what kind of cleanser you use will depend on your skin-type - and exfoliate; that is, you make sure you have removed all the dead cells that can build up on the outer layer of skin. You protect the skin from sun damage with a sunscreen during the day and you nourish it at night.

This is the standard mantra relayed by every beauty column. But I spotted two gaps in the sun protection offered by this routine. Sunscreens do not survive washing and toweling, so the average woman has no protection from the moment she leaves the bathroom at night until she puts moisturizer on her face the next day - whatever hour that happens to be. The other problem is that nearly everyone does not use enough of either moisturizers or sun protection creams to provide day-long protection. They tend to scrimp when it comes to putting cream on the skin.

Dr. Russo's skincare range

As a cosmetic dermatological surgeon (one who treats conditions that affect the skin), I have been made acutely aware of the harm that sun exposure inflicts on the skin of my patients every day. Up to 80 percent of premature ageing can be blamed upon sun damage. So I have developed a range of anti-ageing skincare products based on these simple principles. If you use my scientifically formulated cosmeceutical range correctly, at the right time and in the right quantity, you will avoid premature ageing and you will, in effect, become my patient.

I have devised a way to incorporate a sunscreen into a cleansing lotion. A sunscreen contains a chemical that absorbs the energy of the ultraviolet light, thereby protecting the skin, and its strength, that is its capacity to shield the skin, is represented by a sun protection factor (SPF): the higher the SPF, the greater the protection. Correctly applied, a cream containing SPF 30 should protect the skin from 98 percent of light damage. Sunscreens higher than this offer only minimally added benefit. If you use my skincare products, daytime moisturizer and cleanser, in the quantity recommended, your skin will be protected not only in the day, but at night and in the early morning when it may be light for some time before you go through your skincare routine.

What is *cosmeceutical* skincare?

You can see that this name is made up of two words - 'cosmetic' and 'pharmaceutical'. This means that the product works to improve your appearance (cosmetic) and that it works pharmaceutically, through active chemical ingredients. In practical terms, it means that you can buy it over the counter, without a prescription, as with other cosmetic products, but that it contains compounds with tested drug-like actions and benefits. Cosmeceutical ranges are usually formulated by qualified dermatologists and physicians. In common with the drugs you swallow, cosmeceuticals must undergo testing to demonstrate they deliver what they promise.

The active ingredients in a cosmeceutical product might be an antioxidant (eliminates harmful free radicals), phytochemical (chemicals based on plants), enzyme (a chemical that cause a reaction), and/or essential oils. In order to be effective, these ingredients must remain stable even when the cream or lotion they are contained in has been exposed to air during use. They must also be present in sufficient concentration to produce the desired result. For example, ascorbic acid generally doesn't work if there is less than 10 percent in a cream. Ascorbic acid also reacts with the oxygen once it is exposed to air, so it has to be bound into the cream during the manufacturing process to retain its potency. These considerations, along with making the cream feel and smell nice are factors cosmetic designers have to master before they present it to the public.

Here are some of the active ingredients that are used for cosmeceutical products, many of which I have employed in making my skincare range:

Alpha Hydroxy Acids (AHAs)

AHAs like glycolic, maleic, and lactic acids speed up the skin's exfoliation process, preparing it for active treatment products. They are also the active ingredients in a number of rejuvenation treatments.

Antioxidants

Ascorbic acid (vitamin C), vitamin E, green tea and idebenone stimulate the growth of new collagen and are also anti-inflammatory.

Botanicals or phytochemicals

Compounds like kinetin derived from plants improve light-damaged skin and are less likely to irritate sensitive skin.

Dimethylaminoethanol (DMAE)

A naturally occurring substance that can be taken by mouth as well as applied to the skin and which helps tighten skin and reduce facial sag.

Enzymes
Plant enzymes like papain (found in paw-paw) or pineapple, eat dead skin cells.

Epidermal Growth Factors (EPG)
These counteract loss of skin elasticity and discoloration.

Hormones
Natural (plant) progesterone helps to counteract flushing and redness due to the menopause or the skin condition rosacea.

Niacinamide
Part of the Vitamin B Complex, evens out skin tone and is anti-inflammatory.

Peptides
Copper peptides and argireline reduce wrinkles, smooth and soften the skin.

Four essential elements

There are essentially four elements to my skincare range:

1/ Cleanser, which uniquely for a cleanser incorporates a SPF that remains on the skin after washing
2/ Night exfoliant
3/ Day moisturizer
4/ Night serum (skin-food) and I've thrown in an extra night serum especially for the eyes

Each element comes in formulations to suit either normal to oily or mature skin types. I hope to also introduce a shaving cream that incorporates a sunscreen because many men don't wear moisturizer, although it would be a good idea if they did.

Cleansing and exfoliating: The skin is the largest organ in your body. It is the barrier between the inner you and the outside world. It keeps important things in like moisture and natural oils, and harmful things out, such as polluting fumes, smoke, heat, cold, and sunlight. Your skin is also a processing organ; it produces oil, sweat and impurities. This is why it has to be regularly cleansed; otherwise the impurities that the skin has expelled may build up and clog the pores causing blackheads, pimples or acne. Normally the cells in the outer layer of the skin renew themselves every 28 days. But environmental factors, lifestyle, diet, and the time of year may cause the process to slow down, increasing the build-up of dead cells and making the skin look dull, grey, rough and lifeless. This is why we need to slough off these dead cells (exfoliate) every day with either mechanical (those slightly granular skin rubs) or chemical exfoliants.

My cleanser for normal to oily skin contains active antioxidant cleansing ingredients, plus anti-inflammatory, antiseptic and anti-acne ingredients (especially important for oily skins which are prone to pimples and acne). In addition, my cleansers also release SPF, which adds to the SPF protection provided by the daytime moisturizer. It's important to use the cleanser in the quantities recommended. The version for more mature or sun damaged skin includes pigment lightening and exfoliant ingredients.

Protective moisturizer: To avoid the premature ageing caused by light exposure, the skin must be protected from the ultraviolet wavelengths of light, UVA and UVB. The ideal daytime moisturizer contains SPF 30, as mine does.

I make no apology for returning to the importance of using the right quantity of skin products. Scientific studies done by the American Academy of Dermatology have shown that the average person does not put enough sunscreen on the face. The American Food and Drug Administration (FDA) recommend that 1,000 micro-liters be applied per 50 square centimeters of skin. What does this mean in real life terms? The average adult face has an area equal to a piece of copy paper. (It isn't very easy to drape copy paper over your face, so please take my word for it.) This translates into about 810/820 square centimeters, which means that you would need about 1.6 centiliters (0.016 liters) of sunscreen to protect your face adequately. A teaspoon equals 5cc or one-sixteenth fluid oz. so if, to play safe and allow for the small bits of cream that remain on your fingers, you apply half a teaspoonful, you're probably safe. Most people use less than half this quantity.

Most of us don't measure out face cream with teaspoons, let alone in carefully calculated centiliters and most sunscreen lotions and face creams don't come with specific instructions, or the directions on their labels are just too vague. Clearly what is needed is a sunscreen that works at the small densities most people spread cream on their faces, and for the creams to come in a pack that explains how to apply the correct amount. If in addition this cream gives the face a pleasantly 'tanned' appearance, this should encourage people to use it rather than risk getting a tan by going into the sun. This is how I have made my moisturizer.

The sunscreen ingredients in my moisturizer include physical and chemical filters like titanium D. (that's the white lipstick you may have seen people wearing in the sun), zinc O, avobenzone, octinoxate, tinosorb, and mexoryl SX. If you want the full scientific low-down on sunscreens you can find it well explained at http://www.iranderma.com/text1.htm.

But there is another problem about sunlight. Even when your skin is protected by a generous layer of sunscreen nearly half the harmful free radicals produced by UVA can still get through to damage the skin. This is why we have added active antioxidant and anti-inflammatory ingredients to the sunscreen filters. Vitamins C and E have also been shown to provide protection against UVA and UVB light. I am explaining the science so that you can appreciate the thought that has gone into this range, but, as they say, "the proof of the pudding is in the eating". There is no substitute for seeing how a product performs on your own skin.

Repairing night serum with antioxidants. The best time to nourish and restore your skin is at night, while you sleep. At night the skin has no need to defend itself from environmental onslaughts like sun, smoke, wind or carbon monoxide fumes, but is free to take some well-earned R&R and to concentrate on cell renewal. My night serum contains a complex of antioxidants and active moisturizing ingredients. The version for oily, acne-prone skin is fortified with anti-inflammatory, antiseptic and anti-acne ingredients, and the one for mature or sun damaged skin contains pigment-lightening and exfoliant ingredients. Use the night serum generously and let it work while you sleep.

What about 'nutriceuticals'?

The term 'nutriceutical' is a combination of 'nutrient' and 'pharmaceutical'. It has been used recently in two ways: to describe work of plant biologists developing agricultural foods that are engineered to carry a payload of some beneficial additive. This could be a vitamin or a helpful drug, like the recent announcement of a purple tomato that had been engineered to contain large quantities of antioxidants that could protect against cancer.

But the word is also being applied to a variety of non-prescription products promoted as enhancing health, and by association, health and beauty. These products are usually naturally occurring substances (vitamins, amino acids, herbal products) or formulations incorporating these substances. This kind of nutriceutical is part of the mushrooming market for dietary supplements or 'superfoods'. Their aim is to increase health (and beauty), rather than correct a deficiency or ease some medical problem. Several 'beauty foods' are on sale. There is a ready-to-drink tea (rich in flavonoids) and yoghurt (contains zinc and calcium which are good for nails, clearing up blemishes and even combating brittle-bone disease.)

While this is true in general terms, if a doctor tells you that you have osteoporosis, or brittle bones, you would be wise to take something more powerful than yoghurt to treat it. According to the on-line Euromonitor International, we are even promised a tea-based skincare drink from a major cola company not commonly associated with healthy food, and an anti-ageing jam. 'Chocolate could also become a key beauty sector; rich in antioxidants, the food industry has already put a lot of work into repositioning this guilty pleasure as healthy,' says the site. Like blueberries, another 'superfood', these foods certainly contain health-promoting ingredients and are a sensible part of anyone's diet, though it is virtually impossible to prove precisely how much more healthy or beautiful they will make you.

Analyzing the unique DNA composition of your skin

You have probably heard of DNA. DNA is sometimes described as the basic building blocks that make up a living thing - animal, human, plant - and which also contains the information to make another generation of animal, human or plant modeled on the same lines as the parent. The DNA of all human beings is 99.9 percent identical. But it is that tiny, vital 0.1 percent that makes every human being different and unique. (Scientists have discovered minuscule differences in the DNA of identical twins who used to be thought to be 100 percent the same).

In recent years, scientists have learned how to unravel the DNA make-up of animals, plants and human beings. This is being used to identify criminals by the tiny traces they leave at the scene of a crime. It is also being used to develop new, custom-built drugs and tests for disease, because those tiny little differences in our DNA make some of us more inclined to develop an illness, to respond to drugs or get side-effects with them.

The makers of skincare products are now experimenting with something similar: customized skincare creams. Skin varies from person to person; it is more or less sensitive to light, how rapidly is repairs itself, how well it protects itself from the various harmful substances in the environment. There are reports that some beauty clinics are offering customized skincare products. They first take a swab from inside the cheek (using those extra-long Q-tips you've seen on TV) and send this off to a lab to read that person's unique DNA. The ideal ingredients are then assembled to match that individual's skin profile. It is an attractive, if expensive idea and the journalists that reported on DNA-analysis creams liked them, though they do not produce the sort of dramatic results that make good before and after photographs.

CHAPTER 8
Looking at the future

"You're not going to take somebody who is 60 and turn them into a 20-year-old, but it is very clear that you can take people's skin and make them look younger and more vibrant."

David Goldberg, Director of Skin Laser & Surgery Specialists, New York & New Jersey.

The pace of scientific discovery has galloped ahead in the past 80 years. There have been as many important discoveries in that time as in all the years leading up to it. And the signs are that we will go on progressing by leaps and bounds. What does the future hold for rejuvenation therapy? Judging from the progress we have made in the last decade, a great deal. I first became interested in what could be done to combat skin ageing because I was so fascinated by the way an unborn baby's skin healed without a scar. We now know that some of the amazing physical processes that enable a baby to grow from a tiny group of cells and to differentiate into the specialist blood, bone, muscle brain and fat cells that go to make up a complex, fully-developed adult, are still present in that adult's body. They contribute to the body's capacity for self-repair in the face of certain forms of damage, and they have the potential to repair the body in exactly the same way they do in the unborn baby. It even looks as if they may ultimately enable us to repair and regenerate diseased and damaged parts of the adult body.

"...stem-cell therapy could augment the human body's own regenerative capacity, which declines as we grow older."

Nadia Rosenthal, stem cell researcher.

You have probably heard of stem cells. They are the chameleons of the cell family. We call them *pluripotent* stem cells, because they have the power to become many different sorts of cell and therefore to regenerate or repair every part of the body depending on how they are programmed. They carry the promise of miracle cures for age-related illnesses like heart disease or terrible injuries like a broken spine. Nadia Rosenthal of the European Molecular Biology Organisation believes that in a few decades improved understanding of stem cells could lead to 'disease prevention and life extension.' Studies of mice suggest that the age-related decline in the rate at which parts of the body, like skin, bone or hair regenerate could be reversed, and that one day stem cells may be used to rescue damaged or ageing tissues. If and when this day comes the effects will inevitably be far superior to what we can currently achieve in the rejuvenation clinic.

There are still many questions to answer about the role of stem cells. There is the important issue of where they are obtained. The most versatile stem cells are those recovered from an unborn baby (a fetus or embryo) or from the umbilical cord of a baby. These are called *embryonic* stem cells, but these are inevitably in short supply and collecting them is surrounded by ethical problems. But they are also present in an adult human body, though it is more difficult to extract them. If they are taken from an individual they are called *autologous*, meaning 'from yourself' as an adult, as opposed to those only found in immature tissue. In the adult they may be found in the marrow of the bone and are used to treat some forms of cancer or even, for example in a pioneering German clinic in Cologne, to repair damaged hearts.

The US Food and Drug Administration recently approved the first experimental use of a technique called Cytori Celution for serious medical conditions. This is unique in that stem cells are extracted from the patient's own fat cells, and extraction and use take place at the same time and during the same procedure. (With bone-marrow stem cells they are extracted, processed and stored prior to use). A small number of patients have been enrolled in a fully-controlled medical trial to test whether the technique will be safe and effective in the treatment of heart disease. This treatment is the most advanced application of Cytori technology, but something similar specially designed for cosmetic and reconstructive surgery is already available in Europe and Asia. So to some extent this it is not the future we are talking about here, but tomorrow

You may be thinking that we have talked elsewhere about using the patient's own, that is autologous, fat in rejuvenation therapy. That is perfectly true. The difference in the Cytori technique is that the stem-cells are extracted from the fat, and the presence of the stem cells enables a network of blood vessels to be established (called vascularization) at the site where they are placed to achieve repair. The reason ordinary fat cells are, over time, reabsorbed by the body when they are used for rejuvenation implants, is that they do not set up this all-important blood supply. Where skin cells are concerned, the day-to-day business of replacement and repair slows down in old age. It is possible that by harvesting and implanting autologous stem cells, that this decline could be halted or even reversed.

Hope for baldness

A number of researchers are on the verge of finding a cure for baldness. Last summer, a conference of leading hair-replacement surgeons in Rome heard research into what is called 'follicular cell implantation' - the follicle is the little pocket under your scalp where hair is grown. This has been carried out by a British team backed by a £1.9 million ($3 million) government grant and had yielded 'positive results on human beings'. The process is also known as hair cloning - something you've probably heard about in the context of sheep, other domestic animals and pets. The idea of cloning hair has been around for some years, but Intercytex, the company behind this research claims that they now have a treatment that will work for more than 60 percent of patients after only six months, and for an even greater proportion, if the scalp is first stimulated by gentle abrasion that encourages hair growth. This percentage was based on a very small number of patients in the initial trial, but it is certainly encouraging for all those who have lost their hair through burns, cancer treatment or advancing age.

Hair transplanting, the common current treatment for baldness, takes strips of hair containing healthy hair follicles from the back of the scalp where growth tends to persist even when over the rest of the head it has given up and transplants them to a bald area. It is time consuming and uncomfortable, scars the back of the scalp, and there are limits to how many strips can be transplanted. Hair cloning also harvests productive hair growth cells from the back of the patient's scalp, but then persuades them to multiply many times over by immersing them in a special, patented culture before injecting them back into the scalp in their millions to stimulate the formation of new productive hair follicles, or to rejuvenate those that have given up over the rest of the head. More than a thousand tiny injections may be required to achieve a satisfactory effect. 'Hair surgeons and their patients have been waiting for something like this since the 1980s but in my view, it may be as little as five years before patients start seeing the benefits,' said Bessam Farjo, one of those conducting the trial. Experts at the Rome conference welcomed these early findings with cautious enthusiasm. 'If they really have done this then that is quite an achievement, but I would like to see all the data,' said one prominent Dermatologist.

In the misty distance

Doctors are naturally cautious people. Newspapers may be fond of 'Miracle wonder drug' headlines, but those in the business know that most medical advances progress by small steps, and that for every three steps forward there will probably be one step back. New treatments are not usually the sensation that is at first proclaimed; fewer people may benefit than had been hoped; the side effects of treatment may turn out to be more severe or more widespread.

Nevertheless, I am going to do something uncharacteristic for a medical doctor; I am going to stick my neck out and say that in my view, within a decade open surgery will be virtually a thing of the past. Operations that involve big incisions (cuts), patients knocked out for long periods by risky anesthetics, a great deal of blood loss, heavy scarring, and long hospital stays for recovery will be a rarity. We will probably always have open surgery to repair the damage of road and other accidents, but most medical procedures will be carried out remotely using either natural openings in the human body or small incisions through which special fine tubes and fibre-optic cables will allow the surgeon to see where he is operating and use minute, remote controlled tools to perform the operation.

More and more things will be done under local anesthetic and far more procedures will not even require doctors to go inside the body but will be carried out through the skin using new technologies like ultrasound, X-rays and special wave-length light. It's a brave new world ahead of us and I am convinced the rejuvenation techniques will move ahead in step with these advances. In ten years time or less, I will have to write another book.

CHAPTER 9
Some Leading International Anti-aging Clinics

Mario Luca Russo MD
The Rejuvenation Clinic,
43 Devonshire Street, London W1 G 7AL
Tel: +44 0870 243 2230

and

Canada Place Mall, Canary Warf, London
Tel: +44 0870 243 2230

www.rejuvenationclinic.co.uk

Tina Alster MD
The Washington Institute of Dermatologic Laser Surgery,
1430 K Street, NW,
Suite 200, Washington, DC 20007
Tel: 202-628-8855

www.skinlaser.com

Jean Carruthers MD
740 - 943 W Broadway, Vancouver, BC V5Z 4E1
Tel: +1 604-730-6133

www.carruthers.net

Patricia Wexler MD
Wexler Dermatology,
145 E 32nd St, Floor 7, New York, NY 10016
Tel: 212-684-2626

www.wexlermd.com

Jean Louis Sebagh, médecin
(home)
64, Rue Longchamp, 75116 Paris
Tel: +33 1 47 04 65 75

www.drsebagh.com

and

(practice)
The BA Institute, 64 Knightsbridge,
London SW1X 7JF
Tel: +44 207 351 2040

www.ba-institute.com